DESPERATE TIMES

LINDY KATO

N & I Press

A catalogue record for this book is available from the National Library of New Zealand.

Soft Cover ISBN: 978-0-473-75615-4

Cover design by Rhi Creations

Cover from personal photograph

Edited by Lesley Marshall of Editline

This memoir is a personal account based on real events. It has been necessary to obscure names of family, friends, patients and colleagues throughout for moral and privacy reasons. Material is based on personal recall which come mostly as videos – uninvited and incessant. Have they degraded with constant replay? I have no way of knowing, but every effort has been made to verify accuracy where possible. I apologise for any omissions in this respect and will be pleased to make the appropriate updates in any future edition.

For Dad who wanted to be sure I had an education so I could pay my way in the world since I was too feisty to find a husband.

For my Sweetheart who has proven him wrong over the last forty-five years and is in it for the long-haul.

Without either of you in my life this would not have been possible.

Contents

Chapter 1: Desperate Times

London, England, August 1979

I am pushed out of a moving train. It is an accident – I am certain. What happens next is callous and deliberate.

With my stomach pressed hard against the central pillar of the station steps, I feel a thousand commuters kick and stomp me. Someone trips over my prone torso and lands face first on the concrete. They swear at me! No one is stopping to help. The trampling can only have lasted for a matter of minutes, but it felt longer. I'm alone, pinned at the Coopers Row exit, alive but too stunned to move.

There is a mass of blood on the concrete, but nothing feels broken. Astonishing, because my forty-six-kilogram frame has barely any padding. My lucky charm bracelet has punctured holes around my wrist, staining my white Afghan coat a dirty pink where the coat and blood have mixed with the filth from the platform. "Afghan" is the fashionable term for a thick sheepskin; it must have protected me from the initial impact with the platform, and by absorbing some of the kicks.

I usually take the crowded District line tube train which stops at fourteen stations between Dagenham Heathway and Tower Hill, but this morning I fancied a walk in the early sun and caught the faster overground train that stops only once between Dagenham Dock and Fenchurch Street. It easily makes up for the longer walk to the station and it should have been the healthy option!

By the time any train reaches Dagenham I expect to be squeezed in and inhale someone else's breath. Happily, I got jammed facing the door. As we approached Fenchurch Street, an arm extended around my waist and took hold of the latch. This is a common ploy for a quick exit; it gives a commuter the edge in the race to the ticket collector.

The train jolted, and the arm lurched forward, simultaneously letting the latch go. The door flew open with the platform still a few metres away and the passenger behind

1

(presumably the latch holder) fell against me, pushing me out. I hit the leading edge of the concrete, already horizontal and rolling – akin to a sausage wrapped in sheepskin pastry – until I was halted by the central pillar of the steps. Possibly my twig legs didn't even hit the platform, held high by the bulk of the coat.

I haul myself up the post. Taking the Coopers Row exit I stagger around the corner to Tower Hill.

Education was supposed to be my ticket out of the working class. You can marry your way out, but Dad decided early on that it wasn't likely, so he made sure I got into the "A" class. Officially our primary school wasn't streamed. Amazing, then, that every year the "A" class kids all passed the eleven-plus – essential for any kind of academic qualification. The rest of the year would all fail, bar the odd – and I mean odd – few. The country needs more factory workers, typists and shop girls than it does smarty-pants. I might have fallen into the odd category, but Dad wanted certainty. He had leverage on his side. The school had tried to teach my brother for the best part of three years without noticing he was stone deaf; he was backwards they'd said! I am sort of estranged from my parents, which I don't want to think about.

I passed the eleven-plus. There was nothing mysterious about it because we practised most days. I won a scholarship to a posh school, then got thrown out a few years later. I don't have qualifications for university entry, but my seven O-levels demonstrate that I am trainable. The school wasn't set up to train office girls. Their brochure made a big deal of the fact they didn't offer typing as a subject. An unfathomably large number of students went on to be accountants, some went into teaching, some medicine. All my old school chums are professionals, which was exactly what Dad wanted. My final school report said, *Lindy is a waste of oxygen.* Quite harsh, I feel.

I am a temporary office worker for hire via an agency. It is only one step up from general dogsbody. The other English girls are often surly, arms folded and complaining about their placement for the day. The woman who allocates the jobs can't be bothered with them. The girls from New Zealand always get hired first and it isn't just because of their cool accent. If a permanent job comes up, the Kiwi girl will get it, even if she can't do it, because of the can-do attitude. I adopted their philosophy. Because of my snobby school I couldn't type, had no shorthand and couldn't operate a switchboard. Sometimes I sat up all night teaching myself how to work this or that. I told the agency I could do anything, and I have had a job every day. Some companies even ask for me by name.

The pay isn't bad, but temping isn't safe – I often work late and travel home alone. One of my old Clearing House colleagues got beaten close to death outside Tower Hill Station. He could do one-arm push-ups and pick up a cigarette lighter in his teeth, yet his strength didn't help him that day. I can't fight my way out of a paper bag. He was supposed to marry a girl who works for Cadbury on the day after the office Christmas function where he threatened to throw his unused wedding ring into the Thames. I ended up buying the ring and got it resized at a Hatton Gardens jeweller. They polished off the bark-like patten and would have collected the excess gold dust and charged me for a service I didn't ask for. My sweetheart isn't bothered by the ring's provenance, but I am reminded of the robbing jeweller every time I see its shiny surface.

I step from the platform, paying careful attention as the guard bawls "Mind the gap." The carriage is completely deserted. I ignore the tube-car advertising panels. Ordinarily I would look out for the Mensa adverts, enjoying their devious quizzes; I'm wasted as an office temp.

The carriage might be empty, but the stench of body odour, cigarettes and spearmint makes me want to vomit. Chewing gum is a horrible habit and why anyone thinks their fag breath will be masked by it is a mystery. I usually sit in the guard's carriage, supposedly safer, but I don't want to explain myself to anyone. My face is wet from tears mixed with blood. Is my head bleeding or is it coming from my wrist where I keep brushing hair out of my eyes? At least my jeans are intact – the good-quality denim was worth the investment. I'm shaking, huddled in the corner of the double front-facing seat and no one has dared sit opposite – I make sure by pretending to be drunk. I look like I will throw up at any moment.

Dagenham Heathway Station is on a shopping strip perpetually "under construction". Every day the builders either wolf-whistle or sing the Bowie cover of "Sorrow" as I go past. They never seem to work, their beer bellies seeping through the holes in their string vests while they sit in the sun and smoke. Usually I shout back "In your dreams!" but today I scuttle past.

I'm left wondering – when did people get fat? In primary school no one was fat. There was a single fat girl in my secondary school class, and only one other in the other five classes making up our year. They were fat at eleven and still fat when I got ejected at fifteen. Nearly a decade ago the builders at our school were lean. Fat glistening with sweat and squeezing through a string vest of a Dagenham builder is a vista that cannot be forgotten.

Why do people piss in phone boxes? I'm holding the door open with my foot while I fish around in my purse for some coins. I tell the flippant young girl on the temp agency switchboard that I quit. She puts me through to the woman who allocates the jobs, and she is not at all sympathetic – in fact outraged would be a fair description. Feeling even worse, I drag my sorry arse home.

Fang the wonder cat runs to the door when he hears my key in the lock. All the people who live in the house train him to do tricks. Fang can open the glass doors to the cabinet and even cardboard boxes to get his beloved furry green ring. Will he miss the attention when Stan and I move? We are about to start mortgage repayments, yet I've just quit my job. Plus, we have a do-it-yourself wedding and cheap-as-chips honeymoon to pay for.

The house is a tip; it always is. My room's not so bad – each of the housemates tend to keep their own rooms in reasonable shape and ignore the shared parts. Fang, my fiancé Stan and I share the room with his complete, but dismantled, motorbike – a Norton 750 Commando Fastback. The crankcase off the bike is being used as a litter tray for the cat. Housemates plus friends are often crammed together in the lounge because we can't heat the whole house, so the lounge is a relatively clean mess.

The kitchen is different; you risk contracting seventeen different sorts of disease if you open our fridge. It is so bad that when we were burgled the only thing stolen was the back door. To reach it the burglar would have gone through the back garden past the motorbike in the shopping trolley (in bits to be fair) and it's a shame he didn't steal the trolley bike because it belongs to a housemate's friend. It does nothing but add clutter to the disaster of a garden. The friend lost his spleen when he crashed the thing, so I feel a bit sorry for him; not too sorry though because he is a liar. The guy used to reckon he rode with the Mongrel Mob and Black Power in New Zealand, and I find two big flaws in his story. Firstly, I don't know much about gangs, but I suspect you ride with one, not swap about. Secondly – presuming he even went to New Zealand, which I doubt – the gang members would have noticed he was Posh with a capital P, and I don't think gangs anywhere welcome posh white boys. Anyway, our burglar took the back door and nothing else. He probably wasn't game to brave the kitchen! When we complained about the house now being even colder, our dodgy Nigerian landlord replaced the door with one from the tip. Uncle Olu gets letters from the Nigerian police – he says his brother works there but I think they are after him for something.

There are three more motorbikes in the hallway. They used to be parked on the illegally concreted front garden beneath the bay window of our upstairs bedroom, but the cracks on each side of the bay are big enough for snowflakes to flurry through so we thought the whole thing might drop off and crush the bikes. Never wanting to spend money on the house, Uncle Olu thinks the bay is fine. Parking our bikes in the hallway is a compromise.

I need to inspect the damage to my face so I skirt around the hallway bikes and head upstairs to the bathroom. It looks worse than it is. I won't get much sympathy without broken bones; all I have is a perforated wrist and no job.

But the housemates are sympathetic. A motley crew we are. Todd and Bevan are brothers, one upstairs and one downstairs. They are responsible for two of the hallway bikes; the third is my cherished Honda 400 Four. The downstairs brother hasn't been out of bed for months. We even visited his parents, hoping they would try to extract him. He is horribly pasty and has the curtains shut all the time. In my mind curtains are only closed in the daytime due to a death. I believe Bevan is functionally dead, even if not ready for burial. Then there's Stan and me, and lastly Neil, the token hippy with waist-length hair, who lives in the boxroom. He doesn't have a motorbike, but he does have an ultraviolet light, so the room is weirdly lit and every speck of dandruff shows up. We all get along well, the rent is paid on time, and I am sad to be moving, but it's time to go.

There isn't time to think about finding a job. We rebuild the Norton and then find we have to remove the bannisters to get the thing down the stairs. Even though the house is a mess I want my room spotless since Neil is moving in, though I suspect his black light will kill anything I don't! An ex-boyfriend of mine is taking the boxroom; the less said about him the better. Stan is endlessly patient and quite grown up. He's quiet about the job issue but cares about the train problem. We can hang on with one income for a couple of weeks, not more than that.

My perforated wrist has healed by moving day but now I am struck down with chicken pox. Neither of us has a car licence so a friend hires the moving truck. All I can do is lie amongst the boxes and try not to scratch the pustules.

With the truck unloaded and pustules mostly intact, we walk around the tiny garden like landed gentry. We had tried to find something older, with more character. We even thought about an old warehouse along Canary Wharf in London, but realistically banks will only lend to young couples on what you would call a cookie cutter home.

The houses in our estate are all in the same brick with the same, white-painted window frames, and the roofs are a uniform style and colour – there are no fancy bits to soften the look or add privacy. They differ only by the number of bedrooms (three or four), and some are orientated slightly differently. Trees, bushes and fences are not allowed in the front gardens under a line-of-sight bylaw, so drivers have a clear view through the maze of roads all named after poets. Unusually this estate has a little square car park and along one side is a medical centre, a butcher, a bijou supermarket, and an off licence. The pub is a bit over a mile away but there isn't a church – astonishing for England where pubs and churches appear to go hand in hand.

The location is better suited to our price bracket but not great for work. Working in London is only feasible by train. You can't park a car in London, and I can't drive. Last year the company I was working for bought an annual train pass on my behalf and I was paying them back by instalments but, in need of cash, I sold it back to British Rail. So then I took the Honda each day and on one trip a double decker bus ran over my foot while I was stopped at traffic lights. Another time I came back to my bike late at night to find it had been run over. Which is why I have had to resort to the train again. Even if I wasn't off train travel it is twice as far as it was from Dagenham.

I have never thought about long-term job prospects, always being happy to eat week by week. Things are different with responsibilities.

Scouring the local newspaper, I find four jobs. Office Junior sounds dreadful. Lollipop Man involves hanging out by a busy road in all weathers, escorting recalcitrant children, and is usually a job for pensioners. Waitress? You must be nice to people which counts me out. The only job left is for a Girl Friday. Reluctantly, I apply. They give me an interview, but it is more of a cursory glance to see if I'm tidy enough. Girl Friday, it transpires, is a trendy term for a typist. I am sacked on day three. That will be because I can't type.

Scanning the paper once more, I notice an ad for temporary factory work. This would be Dad's worst nightmare come to fruition. They make stereos, and because of the Christmas rush they need extra employees for three months. Surely, I could manage three months? I would have time to think about my future. Plenty of time, I should imagine – factory work can't be all that demanding.

They don't even bother to interview me; a pulse is the only requirement – though looking around I'm not sure about that. The factory has a contract from the bona fide manufacturers for Sony, who have been unable to keep up with demand. This place usually does very low-end stuff. I will be building the final product from components made here. Then the completed stereo will be sent to the original company who will send it to Sony. I am certain Sony will never know it was made by a third party! Even a cursory glance tells me this is not a preferred contractor.

I have to solder components into the casing; Karen shows me how. The work is fiddly and I'm slow. Tea break and lunch is strictly timed and I'm on my feet all day. By the end of the first week I'm in the firing line. I should be able to put at least sixteen of these things together in a day; I can do eight at best. Karen can do around twenty. She is the boss of me but she's as thick as two short planks. She says to glue where it is too hard to solder. I am conflicted. I cannot resort to glue because the stereos won't work, yet I'm here for a short time, so I have no intention of having it out with her. She can only see that she is the star employee, and I am the one in trouble.

I get shifted to heat sinks. I'm supposed to solder a heat sink onto a tiny component every seven seconds. If I take too long the heat sink will blow – that is their point. I should be able to do five hundred in an hour, but I am hopeless. The fumes sting my eyes and my head pounds. This job is so boring I can't focus; by the end of the week my best hour has only two hundred and fifty that still work.

I get moved to fault finding. If a unit doesn't work when I test it (easily half of them), then my first check is to see what components are glued in! This I can do. The work is relentless. With office work I am used to wandering off, making deliveries, having pub lunches and chatting. Even if chatting were allowed, I have nothing in common with these girls.

Boxes arrive for the Sony goods, and they get piled up on the steps to the only fire escape and stacked against the roller door, which can no longer be opened. Fumes build up within the factory. The girls here are already so limited it won't make any difference, but I am getting brain damage and I'm having fire nightmares. Waking night after night in a panic, unable to escape because of black smoke from burning polystyrene. Polystyrene gives off carbon monoxide, which gets stuck in place of oxygen in the blood. Death by suffocation.

I quit. I haven't even made it to two months.

Snuggling into bed as one of the great unemployed, I can't help but feel glum.

"They are looking for trainee nurses to start in January," Stan announces.

I snort because I choke and laugh at the same time. "I don't make my own bed; I'm certainly not going to make them for other people!" I roll over to spoon with him, his six-foot, wiry frame a perfect carapace for my tiny body.

"Nurses don't only make beds, you know. Desperate times and all that."

Desperate times indeed.

Figure 1. The City Lunatic Asylum, near Dartford. Now known as Stone House.

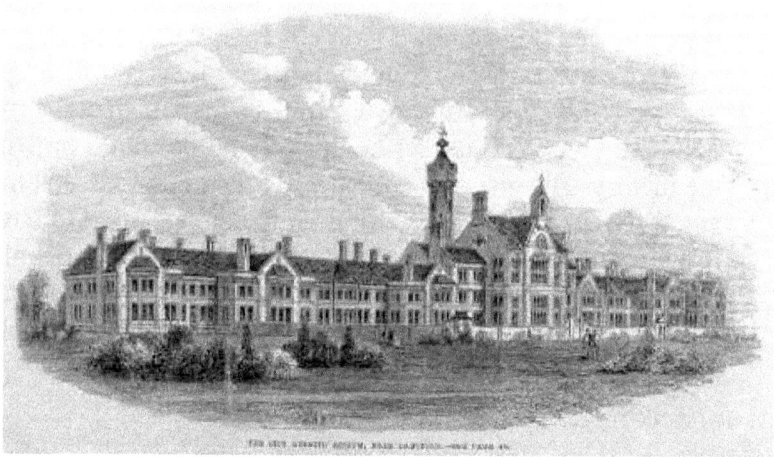

Credit: Wellcome Library, London. Originally published in 1866.

Chapter 2: First Impressions

Turning onto our short sloping driveway and switching off the engine – I heave my left leg over the bike seat like a geriatric and make two unenthusiastic attempts to get the Honda onto the centre-stand before leaving it on the inadequate side-stand. Stan is watching from the doorstep but doesn't rush to help.

"I need a bath, a large glass of port, and bubbles." I put my order in while pulling off my crash helmet. "Bubbles in the bath not the port." Clarity is essential here.

"Was it that bad?" He comes and hauls the bike onto the centre-stand before it rolls backwards.

"Worse!" I stretch my seized muscles. "They had organised a tournament, staff vs patients, I played badminton all day; I can barely stand."

Today was day one of my first proper placement as a student nurse. I consider myself relatively fit, I'm slim, don't smoke and my liquid lunches in London ended when I went temping. Most of my imbibing was done before I was legally old enough to drink. At twenty years and five months, my mad, bad years are behind me, yet I can hardly crawl up the stairs.

Three years of minimal pay whilst training seems like a secure short-term option. I can't imagine psychiatric nursing involves too many bed pans or hospital corners, but I may have walked into a time-limited career. Word has it the loony bins are to be emptied. In fact, the number of people incarcerated has been dropping for a long while, even before the advent of useful medication in the 1950s. Then numbers really began to plummet after Enoch Powell's big speech in 1961.

"If we err, it is our duty to err on the side of ruthlessness.
For the great majority of these establishments there is no,
repeat no, appropriate future use."

Sinking into the bath and using my big toe to add more hot water, I try and rationalise the last few weeks. It has been nothing like I expected. Stan wants to know how you can be paid to play badminton for the best part of eight hours.

"They had pushed the furniture to the edge of the dining room and put up two badminton nets, the courts were a bit small, but it didn't help me, I got thrashed," I tell him. "They are all young and fit and know how to play. I used to play at the youth club, but I was useless then and I don't know the rules. The only break from playing was handover between the shifts and it wasn't even a handover. We had a couple of glasses of wine because the Ward Sister has just got her divorce papers!"

To me, newly married, divorce sounds like a disaster, but she said it represented the finality of a bad decision and a fresh start.

"Then the entire morning shift sodded off to the bar!"

Stan works for the CEGB (Centre of Entertainment, Games and Bingo, also known as the Central Electricity Generating Board), yet he doesn't get to play badminton. He reckons I have all the luck.

"The only lucky thing about it was when a big Irish girl went to the bar with them – if I'd had to play her she would have made minced meat of me!" I lower my face under the bubbles. He takes the hint and goes off to cook dinner. I appreciate he is here though. Since we moved he's had to ride through the Dartford tunnel twice a day. We thought a job would come up at a local power station a lot sooner – it must be wearing him out.

The Irish girl, Oognah, is a pupil nurse – a student in training to be an enrolled nurse. Enrolled nurse training is two years – less academic, and less responsibility once qualified. She has a mass of red hair and an overabundance of enthusiasm. She looks like she has been dragged through a hedge and at first I thought she was a patient.

Resurfacing to an empty bathroom, I glug some port from the oversized glass. This is the expensive stuff – the price is the same as all the others but the bottle is half the size. When Enoch Powell swore to empty the loony bins I was two years old and neither knew nor cared. I *do* care that last year the conservative party got into government with Margaret Thatcher as prime minister. Her ambition is to force the closure of the asylums yet back in 1961 she was the guest speaker at the Friern Hospital prizegiving (as MP for Finchley and Friern Barnet, to the north of London not far from Charing Cross) where she declared the English asylums were the best in Europe. She must have been speaking with a forked tongue because she *would* have been involved in Enoch's great closure speech.

The Friern opened in 1851, heralding a new standard of care. Originally named Colney Hatch Lunatic Asylum, it was the largest in Europe and referenced in the *Chronicles of Narnia* as a synonym for madness after the initial high standards of care rapidly deteriorated. Within twenty years there were calls for it to close. Thatcher *will* close the bins, not because there is any "care in the community", the fashionable term for care that doesn't exist, but because the old asylums are too expensive to maintain and on prime real estate. As far as I am aware, The Friern belongs to the Crown and is on seriously valuable land even if the building were to be flattened.

—◦◦—

After I quit the dodgy Sony factory before Christmas I expected to wait months to hear from the nursing school, but I was snapped up – unseen. My student days started straight after New Year. I was given two uniforms – not enough, but because nurses wear their own clothes on the admission wards I won't need them until September, and I may be too fat by then! I was also given a vaccine for tuberculosis (not optional, even though I swear I've already had one).

There are six of us in our intake; it is a small class compared to other classes – three enrolled nurses who are intent on becoming registered nurses, and three complete newbies. Two of the enrolled nurses are male and from Mauritius. They are slightly older than us, the one with a rounded face and thin moustache looks younger than his friend, perhaps because the friend's face is narrow. Then there is Joan, a local enrolled nurse and quite a bit older, I would say. She has an exquisitely manicured, burnished auburn bun, and her clothes are old-fashioned – I mean *old*, forties style, so it's hard to gauge her age. The other two complete rookies are both male and young. Geoff is tall and gangly with a mass of curly brown hair, and he seems younger than me but can't be because you must be at least twenty for psychiatry – they don't take straight from school. Mike is not much taller than me, fair with thick glasses and an accent, Liverpudlian at a guess.

The main training hospital is Stone House, which was opened in 1866, so not long after Colney Hatch as it was then, and with similar high ideals – though care at Colney was already in freefall by then. It is a huge Victorian building set in 140 acres of parkland to the southeast of London in Dartford, Kent. The architecture of the hospital is Tudor Revival and it only took four years to build – which I thought was impressive, but during our introductory tour we were told there was a lot of arguing about it at the time, resulting in a change of building director, and a lot of what we see has been added on over many years. Since World War II it hasn't had much money spent on it. That will be because it was taken over by the National Health Service (NHS) in 1948.

Our guide shows us into a room the size of a ballroom, its ceiling height possibly twenty feet and peeling yellow paint on the walls. The place is empty except for six beds lined up in the middle, each with a yellowed plastic sheet on top of a mottled, pink-plastic-covered mattress and matching plastic pillow. The beds are like custard creams lined side by side but without touching. Each has a wooden box with a big switch and a set of what look like minimal headphones by the bedhead. This is the Electro Convulsive Therapy (ECT) suite. The grounds for wiring people up to the national grid and giving their brains a decent shock of between 70 and 120 volts was the premise that people with epilepsy don't also have schizophrenia. We are told this isn't true, and never was, but what *was* found was people who had depression that wouldn't budge often did well with ECT. Some of these people were so depressed they wouldn't eat, and the treatment saved their lives.

I'm not sure what I think about ECT, but things get even worse when we are ushered into an overly heated, darkened room, and instantly suffocated by a sweet yet rank smell I will never forget; a patient is undergoing insulin shock therapy. Pretty much the reasons for doing this are the same as the one that was never true for ECT. The patient is in a coma which is why we are allowed to gawk. The humid air makes my glasses steam up, but being blind doesn't make things any better. The malodorous air is a mix of sweat and urine. Increasing amounts of insulin are given by injection every day until it induces a coma. The patient stays in a coma for about an hour and then they are given intravenous glucose to bring them round. It all sounds dodgy. The point is to cause a seizure. This is barbaric on any level. Even the registered nurse looking after the patient says this isn't done anymore, and this is absolutely the last person who will have this treatment which is why we are seeing it. We ask each other – why *are* we seeing it then?

I know next to nothing about schizophrenia but I do know about insulin. I passed O-level biology which covered glucose homeostasis, plus I learned about it from one of my aunts (not really an aunt, but a family friend you have to call aunty). Her four-year-old was diagnosed with diabetes and the kid's older sister had to give her insulin injections because Aunty couldn't do it. I also read a ton about it in the school library once I realised it would be better to spend my days surrounded by books than hanging outside the Deputy Head's office.

Insulin is released by the pancreas in response to rising glucose levels in the blood. Glucose can be either used by cells to produce energy or stored as a bunch of glucose molecules stuck together in cells within our liver and muscles. Now called glycogen, it can be summoned back into use for times when you are not eating – for instance while you are asleep. Insulin causes a channel to open in the cell wall to let the glucose in. The beta cells of the pancreas release around 0.25–1.5 units of insulin per hour, so in a day you would release between 6 and 36 units. Insulin therapy patients are given 100 to 150 units a day and sometimes as much as 450 units. This will *seriously* deplete their blood glucose levels, and you can die that way! A few patients got brain damage from the treatment but in some cases this was considered a good thing because it made them less volatile. Sometimes insulin therapy and ECT were combined to make doubly sure patients were cured. I can't imagine they were!

The day after being traumatised by the tour we have a night shift experience. I hang around at home during the day, not able to nap. Once onsite at Stone House we are taken one by one and dropped off at our various wards. My shift is on Female Admission, and I walk straight into trouble. An elderly lady is refusing to take her medication. I can sympathise – in front of her are four giant white pills. Lithium carbonate, the Ward Sister informs me – essential treatment for her manic depression. It isn't my problem; I must watch and learn and do as I am told – I'm not responsible for anything. I disappear into the office to search for the drug in MIMS, the bible of medication. I need to absorb the whole book anyway.

What I read is quite alarming. The stuff is horribly toxic. The old lady arguing with Sister said she usually has one tablet, 400 mg, but now she's been prescribed four tablets: 1,600 mg. This might be OK for someone younger and three times her size, but she is quite right, one tablet would be a correct dose. The standoff between them is becoming heated, but the elderly lady stands her ground. The Ward Sister storms into the office and takes a swig from a hip flask.

Unsure what to do, I ignore the hip flask and decide to have a chat with the old woman. She's white-haired and the size of a sparrow, and I wonder if the prescribing doctor had seen her because MIMS told me toxicity in the elderly is a serious problem. It isn't my place to say anything, yet morally I can't let the Ward Sister bump her off. Luckily I don't need to do anything because the feisty old lady informs me she's going to bed without *any* tablets.

By the time I get back to the office there's a distinct smell of alcohol and Sister is tipsy. Not much I can do so I go to chat with bedtime stragglers. By midnight everyone is tucked up... including Sister. My lunch break is meant to be at 1:00 a.m., so I gently rock her to let her know I'm going. This isn't what I was expecting.

Stone House was extended in 1874, 1878 and 1885, so the place is a rabbit warren. Searching for the boys from Mauritius who are completing their experience in Male Hospital, I get very lost. Joan was sent to Female Hospital, and like them, has to do some actual work, the reasoning being they are already qualified. Mike has gone to Male Admission and Geoff to the admission unit at Mabledon, as observers.

Eventually I find the boys have made themselves comfortable in front of the TV in the patient lounge. With television broadcasting finishing at 1:00 a.m., they are about to start the wet round. This is as glorious as it sounds: they change the sheets on the wet beds, which I am pretty sure is what I said I wasn't having a bar of. I asked them what they knew about lithium. Not much, it turns out – although they've given medication out, they've never had to know anything about it. They left Mauritius to answer the call to arms from a UK Government desperate for nurses, only to discover they were dogsbodies in a country that didn't want them.

They know the Ward Sister is an alcoholic; apparently everyone does. She saw her son hit by a car and killed. I walked slowly back to the opposite end of the hospital deep in thought. Is it helpful to ignore drinking at work? Mind you, in London everyone gets pissed at lunchtime and then goes back to the office. Even I used to have two pints of Guinness for lunch, easily enough for me to be sloshed. Who am I to judge?

—⋀—

I don't mention the drinking when we report back on our night shift experience, but the tutors tell me I was lucky I didn't have to fight about the lithium issue. They agree that 1,600 mg would have been too much for a tiny old lady. They don't give me any answer about how I should have handled it, but we are reminded that we must do as we are told. The new boys were as surprised as me that they essentially did nothing at all

17

during their first experience. The three enrolled nurses with unsupervised placements on the hospital wards were exploited and they knew it. None of us were happy about the visit to the patient undergoing insulin shock therapy. We felt as if we had intruded – it was an archaic barbaric violation, and we were powerless to do anything. We didn't understand the motivation behind sending us there and we didn't get an explanation for it. At least we have two weeks of classroom instruction before reporting for our first placements. There's time to do some research about Mabledon Hospital, my first placement.

Under an 1867 Act, the Metropolitan Asylum Board (MAB) had responsibility for the mentally infirm and for infectious diseases amongst London's paupers. At that time there were regular outbreaks of smallpox. A hospital ship, the *Dreadnought*, had been chartered from the Admiralty and moored in Greenwich to take the overflow from London's hospitals. The *Dreadnought* could take two hundred patients, but then the outbreak abated and the ship was returned to the Admiralty. The use of static ships in the Thames was not unusual – in Dicken's *Great Expectations* Abel Magwitch escaped from a prison ship moored in the Thames, although this was a bit of poetic license because the ship was really moored in the Medway estuary close by.

There was strong opposition to using London hospitals for infectious diseases because of the fear of spread. An outbreak in 1880 caused locals to take MAB to court. This wasn't unreasonable as there was evidence that the closer you lived to a hospital the more likely you were to catch smallpox. A Royal Commission in 1881 claimed it was the state of squalor and a lack of vaccination rather than the hospitals; nevertheless, two hospital ships – the *Atlas* and the *Endymion* – were chartered and moored on the River Thames in Greenwich as before.

Locals were still unhappy with their proximity and so the ships, along with the *Castalia* (a twin-hulled paddle steamer), were moved some twenty kilometres downstream to Long Reach in Kent. Because they were linked together with bridges they were a hazard to other vessels. They were difficult to clean, prone to fire and sometimes delirious patients would throw themselves into the river. The Thames was a sewer and not ideal for sick patients. Long Reach is within the Dartford marsh area and close to the Darenth estate, owned at the time by the Bishop of Rochester.

The land Mabledon Hospital stands on was the original site of a smallpox tent – an emergency solution to overcrowding on the ships that took the less acute patients. When the weather got too cold, as-yet-unoccupied blocks, built to expand the Darenth School for Imbeciles (not my words) – were used. There was a fear for children already at the site, but they were vaccinated and none of them caught smallpox.

As the number of cases grew, several "room" tents were erected on the Mabledon site inside bigger marquee-type tents, housing some three hundred patients and used all year round. Eventually temporary huts, collectively known as Gore Farm Hospital was built in 1890 for convalescing patients and temporary buildings known as Long Reach Hospital and The Orchard in 1902 for the smallpox patients. Joyce Green Hospital opened in 1903. It was closer to the river, so patients didn't have to be transported through the Dartford township, but by then the smallpox problem was all but over, and Joyce Green was used for other contagious diseases. The ships were sold for scrap and the Gore Farm huts became the Mabledon Hospital for displaced Poles. These were mostly WW2 soldiers suffering from shellshock who'd previously been housed near Tunbridge Wells, some fifty kilometres south of Dartford. The thing is, I'm starting my nursing training in 1980 and the Polish refugees are still there!

The Polish part of the hospital is low key; they have a bar, essentially for the Polish patients, though staff use it as well – I'm not sure if they are supposed to! The Acute Admission Ward, where I am to spend six weeks, is unusual in that it is male and female mixed. There is a long ward plus a few double and single rooms. Beds are jiggled to suit the clientele. Acute Admission might sound grand, but it is an old wooden hut with uneven floors and dodgy lino – everything is on the verge of falling completely apart. The whole hospital looks like a series of dilapidated wooden army barracks.

It's the morning after the badminton tournament. A while ago I broke the Honda's kickstart with my forty-six-kilo mass and often it won't start using the electric start, especially in the cold. I end up running along the road, leaping on it, and crash starting it – without actually crashing it. Since I'm still recovering from the badminton there is no way I am capable of the inelegant flying leap today and Stan left early; thankfully, it starts. I'm on some kind of individualised shift covering part of the morning shift and part of the afternoon one. By the time I arrive I feel as if I have been run over by a bus. Looking around, it seems I'm not the only one. Things are very quiet on the unit.

Chapter 3: Blokes and Nights

I am scared shitless creeping from the dimly lit corridor into Male Admission where I will be on night shift for the next eight weeks. Not confident my motorbike will still be in the carpark come morning, I think maybe I should leave now. There is so much history here; the air is palpable. I was scared long before getting this far. When we were shown around the very first week I couldn't help but notice that the men here are overwhelmingly large, somewhat feisty, mostly young and fit, and there are a lot of them. They are here because they are mad, and some of them look really bad.

The Charge Nurse – note, Ward Sister is called Sister, but the male equivalent is Charge. Why is that I wonder? Anyway, Charge introduces me to the lads. He warns them to be on their best behaviour and says they must look out for me. I'm not sure if this helps at all.

Some of them have already turned in. I came in early to meet the evening shift and listen to the handover. This is where the evening staff describe to the two staff on nightshift how the evening has been, but the other nurse has taken leave! I'm here to observe, not fill in for annual leave. After my night on Female Admission, I suppose I shouldn't be surprised. Charge warns me to ignore any advances the men might make, I am twenty, blond and tiny – I am not to be alone with any one patient, but apparently I should be safe enough in a group.

Paul is the scariest looking bloke I have ever seen. His head is square – honestly, he has corners. He is solid muscle, early thirties at a guess. Charge explains Paul is here to give his mother a break. He functions at the level of a twelve-year-old and really should go to Darenth Park, but they can't cope with his behaviour – which includes sexual issues. Paul's mum is on her own. I don't know her, but she must be in her fifties at least. Paul is prone to violent outbursts, and she cannot manage him. She has had to lock herself in her bedroom at times. This is no way for a woman to head into her twilight

21

years. It isn't uncommon for parents to seek respite from their offspring, there are a pair of brothers here for the same reason.

Suddenly office work seems so much more attractive, even if it involves a train. I feel sick and I want to go home.

Nothing happens all night. I am not sure we would know if it did. The dormitory is down some narrow stairs walled each side. The beds are all around the edge of one big room. The head of each bed against the wall and the foot facing the centre, no screening curtains, no privacy at all, yet isolated. It would have to be a big racket or someone coming to tell us before we knew of anything going down. Overnight, everyone went to bed, slept, and in the morning they slowly woke and got on with cleaning teeth and all those mundane things. We write "slept well" on everyone's notes.

The same thing happened Tuesday night, Wednesday and Thursday. Friday was different. The phone rang around 1:00 a.m., so technically Saturday, and it's the police claiming to have two escaped patients. *Escape* must be an exaggeration. There is a back door to the large dormitory. It isn't locked – it can't be, it's the fire door. Once outside, there is a stone wall, about eight feet high, maybe ten, with glass embedded in cement all along the top, but this is a relic from the past because the gates are open. All night and all day. As far as I am aware the only place that's locked, apart from a couple of secure rooms, is where the old folks with dementia are, because they wander.

Charge is taking the call; the police are demanding someone comes to pick them up. Clearly, Charge can't leave me here alone, and I can't drive. Plus, he doesn't believe them. He tells them he will phone them back.

"Never accept anyone at their word," he says. "Always phone back using a number from the phonebook."

This is a lesson; never accept a phone call without first checking they are who they say they are. He looks the station number up in the book. While he does that, he sends me to do a head count. The correct number of bodies and empty beds – two hadn't been occupied. But now those two beds are occupied and two others are empty.

I report back, "We have the right number of bodies, but there has been a bit of bed dancing."

Charge rolls his eyes. "Are they the beds closest to the fire door?"

"Yes."

"Guests," he says.

He is talking to the original police officer again. The boys have said they are dangerous.

"Ooh ooooh, Charge," I interrupt. "The brothers – those are the empty beds."

"OK." Charge carries on with the call. "The choices are, you keep them in the cells, you tell them to walk, or you call a taxi and tell them they will have to pay for it – whatever you like, because we are *not* coming to get them!" He puts the phone carefully back in the receiver.

"So how come we have two extras?" Not an unreasonable question I feel.

"They will have rolled in after the pub shut. Probably a dozen times a year we end up with more bodies in the morning than we started with the night before."

My eyes must have widened as I contemplate why you would stagger into a lunatic asylum and look for a bed. "Does anyone truly say to themselves 'I can't be arsed to walk all the way home, shall I wander around the spooky grounds of the local loony bin and check for unlocked doors in case there are empty beds?' Really, does anyone think that way?"

Charge laughs. "Nothing quite so bizarre – ex-patients know all about the door and a decent chance of finding an empty bed. It will be someone who knows the place and we won't wake a sleeping drunk; we can find out who they are in the morning." Charge is always interested in a quiet life.

We settle down for a game of draughts; he will end up dozing while I do a bit of study. I can't sleep when I'm supposed to stay awake – I find it hard enough to sleep when I should! Then the phone rings again. This time it is the night porter. The reception is closed at night, but the porter informs

Charge that there are two coppers at the front desk with our escaped patients.

I learn this is not the first time this pair have scored a ride home using the police as a taxi service. We will give them a talking to in the morning but now is not the time. We thank the officers and assure them the brothers are not dangerous as they claimed. They will have been to the night club, failed to pick up any hot chicks, or any kind of desperate woman, and decided to cut their losses. Losers rather than crazy axemen.

Like Paul, they are on the ward to give their parents a break, although I have to say Paul has been charming to me. You can see he is doing his best to mind his manners and make a good impression. A pubescent boy type of charm, a bit hit and miss, and over the top. The self-appointed dangerous brothers are very sweet to me as well, they are biological brothers but adopted. Both have been diagnosed with schizophrenia. There is something seriously wrong with the adoption system in the UK. I probably shouldn't say that because I have one adopted cousin who is great. Mum's older sister hadn't managed to conceive, but after adopting a baby went on to have one of her own, which I understand is quite common. There is also an aunt who isn't a real aunty (another one) with an adopted boy, and he seems fine as well. These cousins are children of unmarried ladies who'd got "into trouble", an orphan stream that has mostly dried up.

Another vanished orphan stream are the Chinese babies dumped in Hong Kong. These babies, mostly girls, were left by parents fleeing starvation in China under the rule of Mao Zedong "The Great Leap Forward", a social campaign that ran from 1958 to 1962, was supposed to transform China. Instead it resulted in tens of millions of deaths, and for childless Westerners a source of babies – who were neither orphans nor unwanted. They were dumped in stairwells and stations to be found by strangers in order that they be saved. Technically almost none of these will be orphans because they have at least one living parent. Actual orphans are rare.

There is another, sad stream of orphan babies – those removed from their parents because of alcoholism, drug abuse,

24

or mental health issues. I know a bit about this too because I once had a boyfriend who was a product of this – well, I say "boyfriend" lightly, my brief connection with him could have been a nightmare from which I would never recover.

He was older than me which was important at the time. Having an older boyfriend would surely get me noticed as the sophisticated young woman I was, despite being clumsy and flat chested. We met when he bumped into my table, spilling coffee down my white, cotton smock dress. Quite the disaster for the dress, but his full-on apology and invitation to play table tennis turned me to putty. He looked pretty good, I was only thirteen, and I was flattered.

Next he invited me to Saturday morning pictures. I usually went anyway so if he tagged along it would be OK – my friends might see him.

After the movies he invited me to meet his family and stay for lunch. Everything was turning out better than I'd expected. He said he was adopted, and that it made him chosen instead of being like me, where my parents got landed with whatever turned up. He wasn't wrong because I had already had this out with my parents and Mum had said if I *were* adopted then why would they have chosen such an ungrateful child? He was into art, he said, and he wanted to show me his paintings. It didn't take long to work out that intellectually I was significantly smarter, but appearance was all that mattered to me then.

He took me home and led me to the summerhouse. It makes the place sound posher than it was – a modest bungalow in a nice end of town, a loft extension and a little pond in the smallish back garden – where his clearly intellectually disabled brother was parked – and then the summerhouse. With a bed in it.

I hoped this meant a nap before lunch but I was not totally naïve, and as he lay down next to me I was terrified. He slid his hand down my pants. I froze; whether I was trying to make out I was dead I don't know, and I didn't know about the technicalities of sex either. We hadn't covered it at school.

He tried fiddling about with my girl parts and was getting frustrated. "What's wrong with you?" he said. "Most girls are gagging for it by now."

I managed to ask what "it" might be even though I already knew.

"Sex! We're going to have sex." He sounded astonished that I seemed not to know.

I was a virgin and quite determined to stay that way, and nothing he was doing in my knickers made me think anything different. He got up and stomped off. I wasn't sure what to do next. I wondered if I could slip out, and run away, but his brother would probably see me.

This brother was sitting by the pond, which was an exaggeration – propped up, skinny white arms and legs at odd angles, is more precise. I could see what looked like an adult nappy and a bib to catch his drool. Despite its distortion his face was identical to John's but grotesque rather than attractive. I might have got away without him noticing me leaving but I was brought up to treat everyone with respect.

I reorganised my clothing and opened the door. "Hi, Kevin, did you see where John went?"

Although his head was wobbling, I didn't get any sense he knew I was talking to him.

Then his mum called out to me, "Lunch is almost ready."

I could hardly skip now – she seemed like a grandmotherly type – so I donned my respectful face and offered to help.

She looked relieved, and said she would welcome the help and the company; she never had anyone to talk to. I warmed to her and took over the salad preparation, entirely in my comfort zone – I was trained from the age of five to be boss of the salad. Trying to be polite without being pushy, I asked if the boys were twins. I told her I knew they were adopted and complimented her on how selfless it was of her to take on a disabled child.

She looked directly into my eyes and said, "You aren't like John's usual girlfriends. I have to tell you to stay away from him – he is no good."

I'd worked that out already, but I was surprised to hear her say it.

"We didn't knowingly take on a disabled child. We'd never had a baby of our own and we were desperate. We said we could *not* cope with a disabled child, especially being older parents. Social Welfare didn't tell us. We quickly realised something wasn't quite right about Kevin – he couldn't roll over or hold his head up – but we didn't know much about babies and Social Welfare kept telling us we would make brilliant parents. It's even worse now that he isn't classed as a child; we get no help at all."

I have a cynical streak; although I try and think the best about people, I distrust institutions and their motives.

This lady clearly wanted to talk, and she sounded just like my Nan. It wasn't my intent to intrude but we kept talking.

"Kevin will be a child for our whole lives," she said. "We can't go anywhere and no one comes to visit, but he isn't the biggest problem. John is evil, and we can't get any help there either. He could kill us! You get away from him, dear."

I never saw him again, but a few months after my encounter I read that he'd been arrested after smacking up shop fronts with a golf club. He ended up in a secure hospital diagnosed with schizophrenia.

—∿—

I spend a lot of the nights reading patient notes – they hold a huge amount of information if you dig past the monotony of *slept well* or *passed the day in the sheltered workshop, nothing to report.*

The adopted brothers who used the police as a taxi service have notes detailing a "frigid mother". Their schizophrenia supposedly results from her inability to bond with them. Blame the parents. I suspect the brothers had been removed from crazy parents and inflicted on a perfectly ordinary couple who were then driven to distraction by crazy sons. It also occurs to me that child removal would usually mean some serious neglect or abuse has occurred to the child, and then the removal was likely traumatic too. Children are not removed from loving parents that have brought them up to be well adjusted. Desperate to have children, and only wanting to hear good news, these adoptive parents are suckers being set up to fail.[1]

I am beginning to get a grip on the differences between men and women (I think!). Anxiety and depression don't seem to be common amongst the blokes. Of course, it *could* be rampant but it's not manly to discuss that sort of thing. Men seem to be either mentally challenged and should be in Darenth Park, or they are psychotic. Psychosis is a problem with reality. The title used to cover everything – melancholia, dementia, idiocy – but now specifically has to do with things like hallucinations, disorganised behaviour/thoughts/speech, delusions (beliefs that are demonstrably not true), flat/inappropriate affect, or a feeling of unreality – the list is quite long. A fair few of these patients have had experience with cannabis or LSD (lysergic acid diethylamide). I cannot deny I know quite a bit about that but my friends seem to have come out unscathed.

---

[1] (Nothing has changed see The Guardian Meg Henderson *Adoption Hell* Tue 27 May 2003 09.01 BST)

Chapter 4: Uncle Olu

"Do you know who the bike in the loft belongs to?" Todd is on the phone, and I can tell he is upset. I relay the request to Stan; he shakes his head.

"No idea," I reply. We all know there is a Suzuki Ram Air 380 in the loft plus various other bits and pieces. I imagine someone must know who it belongs to – how can you mislay a bike like that? "Does it matter?"

"The police came. They say we are squatters and have to have everything out by the end of the week. Olu has disappeared."

"Oh, shit, Todd, we're coming over."

No one trusts the police in London, and although Dagenham is on the outskirts it still counts as Greater London. The London cops are a corrupt bunch, so you do have to wonder about the rest of them. The Flying Squad – nothing to do with flying, more a reputation for flying in and clearing up crime – are known as the Sweeney because Sweeney Todd (an errant barber who turned his patrons into pies) rhymes with flying squad, following the simple rhyming slang of London's East End. The boss of the Sweeney is spending eight years in jail. Another twelve cops have also been convicted, and a load more resigned. Things are out of control, so you can't trust a random cop knocking on your door.

My ex now lives in the Dagenham house, known affectionately by its street number, forty-four. He got off in 1976 for an illegal knife he was carrying because a top lawyer claimed the search was illegal, an example of the misuse of the *Sus* law. This refers to section four of the 1824 Vagrancy Act which was intended to prevent begging and fortune telling but is now used for anything, especially if you are young and black. This law requires a police officer to have reason to believe you are acting suspiciously *and* intend to commit an arrest-able offence. My ex isn't black, but I totally wanted him arrested! I found it hard to accept that the court returned the knife. It was an illegal flick-knife, no argument there, but because of the tarnished police reputation the judge was inclined to go with the illegal search scenario.

As an aside, *Sus* is properly italicised because it is the genus name of domestic and wild pigs. Happenstance? I think not.

I put the phone slowly in the receiver, my mind ticking things off, for and against Uncle Olu.

"Stan, we have to go to Forty-four – the police have told the boys to get out and Olu has disappeared. I'm not sure who the crooks are." I never thought I would be defending Olu; I'd always thought the Nigerian police letters were dodgy. If it was his brother, as he claimed, you'd think he would write to Olu's home address not his rental property. He was always friendly though; he came in for a cup of tea and a chat when he collected the weekly rent. We did our best to make sure we had the rent because we didn't want to let him down. On the other hand, he was never keen to spend a single bean on the property.

Taking two motorbikes through the Dartford tunnel would mean paying for both. Besides, the fumes in the tunnel make me dizzy – so much so that if the traffic is stopped I start to hallucinate. Consequently we will both go on Stan's Commando, but I'm not a happy passenger either. I hug him tightly so we move as a single unit.

For the first eight months in our new house he had ridden through the tunnel to work because we had moved so far out to get a place we could afford. We knew it would mean him changing power stations and we thought that would be simple, but a job at a closer station has only just come up, and the shift work he does now is complicating our lives.

In under an hour we are rapping hard on the wooden door, knocking off even more of the blue paint that is suspiciously like the paint used on the roundabouts which seem to be popping up everywhere. The boys can't have gone far – we can see the hallway bikes through the letterbox. No one comes to the door and above us we hear the boxroom window opening. My ex is in the boxroom – everyone starts there – but it isn't him. This is a thin young woman with long blond hair; she could be mistaken for me. She apologises that she can't come to the door, she is locked in. She suggests Bevan might be in. I am certain he is, but he won't, or possibly can't, open the door. Even if his legs would hold him, the outside world would blind him.

As I look up at her she turns into a great white light filling my vision. An iron gauntlet squeezes my heart. I want to scream at her to run but my brain is disconnected from my larynx.

Stan grabs my hand. "They'll be at the pub. Come on."

He hasn't registered the fact that a young woman is locked in a tiny room without a toilet and I can't recall why I am so bothered.

The pub is the *Henry Ford*. We call it *The Pope's Dead* because there was a run of popes when it opened. One died and the replacement lasted barely a month. In fact, the pope's death heralded what has been dubbed the winter of discontent. I don't think the pope had anything to do with it, but the winter of 1978/79 saw practically everyone on strike, notably unions that barely ever went on strike such as health service workers. This was because inflation was so high that pay rises became pay cuts in terms of buying power. The Conservatives got into power because the incumbents were rubbish. There was a stabbing on the night the Henry Ford opened so it isn't salubrious, but it *is* walking distance.

The Ford car factory is on the other side of the busy road via an overbridge. Ford supports most of the community around here – in fact at least a third of my relatives, on both sides of the family, work there. Not my parents, but both have siblings there. The machinists strike of 1968 is what galvanised Dad into fighting for my education. He hadn't thought too much before then, but that strike highlighted the fact that women were paid half what men were. Which was fine if you were married. Well, it was never fine, but people thought it was acceptable – women got written out of wills after finding a husband since they no longer needed the money! But it meant you *had* to get married, and Dad wasn't sure that was achievable. He knew I could never be a homemaker. He didn't want me to work myself to death for half a wage because I wouldn't be able to pay my way in the world. He took the school system on full frontal.

Todd and Dave are in the snug of the Henry Ford. Dave was already living at Forty-four when I moved in – in fact I took his room when he left and I graduated from the boxroom. I need to be sure the guy saying they must get out is a bone fide police officer. Todd says there were two and that they showed their warrant cards, though they were more concerned Olu was hiding out in the house. He is "wanted" now, and immigration are looking for him too. The cops searched Forty-four, but Todd says they didn't rip it apart. They were probably frightened of catching something!

Olu has family; when he came for the rent, he usually tried to sell us something we neither wanted nor needed, but the last time I saw him he bought an old record player of mine that he said it was for his daughter. It wasn't worth much, but he bartered me down to a fiver, trying to make me feel sorry for him and his poor deprived child. The money went straight into the gas meter. The place costs a fortune to heat because of the huge cracks in the walls. Which brings me to the next point.

"So, Olu doesn't own the place he's been collecting the rent for?"

"It's worse than that." Todd takes a large glug of beer for dramatic effect. "The people who own it didn't know it had been let. They are missionaries and have been overseas for years. They rocked up to the house, saw it was occupied, and went straight to the police. They didn't even knock."

"I bet they had a shock when they saw the state of the place. Even without going inside you can see it's gone to rack and ruin. Mostly ruin." Now I don't know who to feel sorriest for.

"I don't want to think about them," Todd replies. "We've been discussing the loft bike. we all thought it was most likely Dave's, but he says it isn't."

Dave is slowly shaking his head.

Todd carries on, "It must be worth a few bob, but now we're worried it's stolen."

I digest this as I go to the bar to get a couple more beers, then I wait for my Guinness to settle. The pub is empty apart from our group of Forty-fours. Stan wasn't really a proper flatmate, but he spent a lot of time there once I moved into the big room. Mostly rebuilding his bike because even with snow coming through the cracks in the walls it was still warmer than the shed at his parents' place. Plus he had been paying half the bills there and we were saving for our house. I would be heartbroken if my little palace was reduced to rubble by a bunch of strangers. Have we been that bad? The house was a wreck when each of us moved in, and none of us knows who Olu rented it to first. We are all too young to afford anything decent. Proper landlords wouldn't rent to us anyway. Todd a courier on a pushbike because he lost his licence, me an office temp before the train incident, and Bevan a dole bludger – though, he *should* be on a sickness benefit. Only Neil has a proper job, on the production line at the Ford factory.

Todd and Bevan will return to their family home. Their mum is sick, they should have gone already. Their Dad won't cope – she is the matriarch in the family.

My ex, wherever he is, will go north to his girlfriend's parents. The Suzuki in the loft predates him anyway. There were never supposed to be two people in the boxroom – realistically it isn't big enough for one. Neil doesn't have anywhere to go, but since he has neither a car nor motorbike, and no desire to drive, he needs to stay close by to get to his job at the Ford works. I take the beers back to the snug and we sit there in the gloom, contemplating.

A sudden shaft of light from the pub door breaks our thoughts, briefly showing up the dust. Neil is so slim the door barely opens as he slips in and it snaps shut behind him. Striding purposefully to the bar, he orders an orange juice and comes directly to the snug without waiting for it.

"I've been to the council offices."

We all look up.

"They say I am *intentionally homeless*." Neil pauses while we take this in, "They say I can go on the waiting list but isn't an emergency. I will never get anywhere on the list, without a family."

He is quite right, single man, with a job, he will stay on the bottom forever. We are all a bit perplexed over this definition of homelessness, considering it involves police and an absentee landlord. Neil says the council are adamant it is his own fault. His plan is to camp on the council lawn in his pup tent. It is coming into summer, but surely, they can't ignore him.

Our attention turns to the state of the place and the excess of motorbikes. Saul can come and get the shopping trolley bike; the hallway bikes will go with their owners.

There have never been any real dodgy dealings at the house. A bit of weed may have been smoked, but not by me – I already came close to frying my brains long before I wound up there. None of us is aware of anything stolen or duplicitous in any way, but no one wants to take the loft bike or the excess bits in case something comes back to bite them. We decide to secure the loft hatch and walk quietly into the distance.

Dave has a driving licence and can hire a truck. Stan and I offer to help but Todd can't see we can be much use without a car (or licence), and he doesn't think it's worth the chance of running into my ex. He has a point.

I hadn't left a single thing there and I'd cleaned my space, and Neil has kept it spotless – I knew he would. We are all responsible for the lounge and kitchen. The bathroom isn't so bad, and the garden was wrecked long before we got there. I guess Todd is right – Stan and I have moved on. Stan has his new job with an extremely confusing shift that includes days, nights, rest days and rolling rest days that we can make neither head nor tail of. I am also on night shift; we are leaving each other written messages and we have learned to date them, otherwise we're never sure what day they refer to. We sup up and say our goodbyes – now we are grown-ups we must get on with our own lives.

—∿—

I have two weeks in the nursing school. The school is a fine old house in the grounds of Darenth Park and what I love the most about it is the huge open fire in the library. You might think it rather dangerous in a library, but there is nothing better than curling up on the carpet in front of a fire. It is hard to drag myself to class. Today, though, as I ride slowly along the magnificent driveway, I notice the fields that last week were yellow – mainly straw yellow, but also some bright yellow of the oilseed rape – are now *smutty* I would call it. Could the ash from the eruption of Mount St Helens last weekend have reached this far?

The eruption was caused by an earthquake, this much I know. I also know people were evacuated. One crusty old soul refused to leave but the death toll (numbers aren't quite in yet) *could* have been in the thousands. It isn't the case because a volcanologist (David Johnston) noticed an increase in seismic activity and persuaded the government to restrict access to the area and evacuate people. He managed to get a call out to say the eruption had started (18th May). He didn't have time to save himself. He died still monitoring activity on the mountain. The seismographs were only installed on the 1st of March and without them this would have been a much bigger disaster. As I survey the fields, I doubt these crops will recover and we are half a world away. I wonder how the rest of the world has fared.

Figure 2. Ectron series 3 electroshock therapy device.

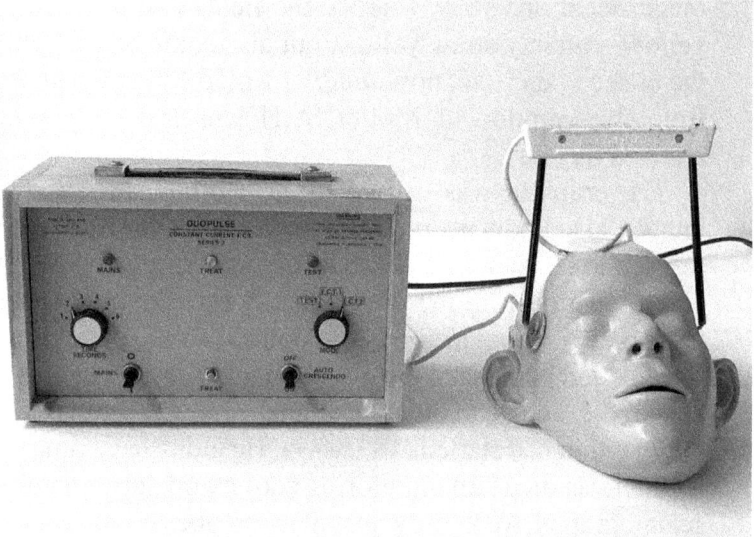

Manufacturers sales photograph circa 1965

Chapter 5: Girls and Nudes

I'm apprehensive as I push through the ornately carved double entry doors for Female Admission. The doors are most likely oak, hidden under thick magnolia paint that is splitting and cracking. I am tempted to slide a screwdriver down one of the splits and peel it all off like plastic sheet. I would if they were mine. My newbies experience in my first week didn't go well on Female Admission. Now, with six months under my belt, I wouldn't say I know what I'm doing, just that I'm less surprised by things that happen. Usually.

It's my second day when Sister receives a call from the hospital shop run by the League of Friends. Patients can get bits and pieces like toothbrushes and newspapers, or have tea and biscuits. Not really a café, more a couple of chairs. There is also a bar which opens in the evenings. Patients can have either two pints of stout or two glasses of sherry. Some of the elderly ladies from the long-stay wards are so tiny two glasses of sherry each night will have them tipsy *every* night. But this isn't a prison and two glasses a night is deemed reasonable alcohol consumption for the average Brit. Of course, I know plenty of people who drink a whole lot more – mostly the staff!

This call, though, is completely different. Oonagh, the Irish girl I met very briefly at Mabledon, is causing some kind of fracas. Sister doesn't elaborate but wants me with her because I know the lass. I assure her I don't, but she insists someone younger will be helpful, considering the situation…

That's all she says, and we leave immediately. There is a Staff Nurse and an Enrolled Nurse left on the ward plus another student. I met the older Ward Sister yesterday, and she seems okay. This one is younger, plump – round, really – and quite sassy. It is hard to believe she is a Ward Sister; they are supposed to be mature (read: old hags). She has already made me laugh out loud, but I can sense her brain running on overtime even though we walk in silence.

I don't know what was said on the phone – but as we round the corner I can't imagine any words that would diplomatically

37

describe the situation. Oonagh is naked and has a rose between her teeth. She is dancing amongst a growing crowd and getting quite exuberant. It is six months since I met her at Mabledon in the badminton tournament. I sensed something was *off* then.

She apparently lives in the nursing home; Sister knows her room number. That fact tells me this isn't entirely out of the blue. Sister is taking Oonagh back to Female Admission and I am to go to her room and get her some clothes.

When I get there, not only is the room unlocked, but it is completely bereft of clothes and furniture. Even some of the wooden trim around the door is missing, the skirting board has gone, and the carpet has been ripped up. It is the end of summer so she can't have burnt the wood to keep warm – how do you lose skirting board?

Back on the ward, Sister has found her a hospital gown. I report my findings and Sister dives into her purse, hands me a tenner and tells me to get her some knickers, a nightie and a toothbrush. She won't be going anywhere for a while. This is more than the hospital shop can provide, and I don't know the area. Walking is going to take too long, so hopefully the bike will start. I should leave it on a slope, but the side-stand is dodgy, and I don't always have the strength to lug it onto the centre stand. Today it is in a reasonable mood; it varies with the climate.

I do my best; she is a big girl but I'm not sure how big. Nightwear should be roomy rather than snug, knickers the same, so I err on the side of *outsized*. When I return Sister is happy, and although she seems to have some kind of relationship with Oonagh, she is arranging for her to be transferred to the Mental Health Unit (MHU) at the nearby Joyce Green Hospital. She thinks they will send her back to Ireland – she says Oonagh came from a remote area and hasn't really coped since she left. Cultural shock, Sister says.

To take stock, there are a lot of people with hallucinations here, but very few take their clothes off. I would say Oonagh's behaviour is at the extreme end of distress. I have had tactile hallucinations myself for many years. Always the same thing – the feeling of hot liquid running down my shins. If my leg was made of pixels then it would start at one pixel and spread. Always down, not radially. It is so compelling, I *must* look. It started in my teens. I was standing in a queue at the bank, and I remember thinking I'd had an unexpected menstruation malfunction – a common teenage angst. But nothing was there. It happens relatively often, but isn't something to mention. It's not that I am used to it – it catches me out every time – but it doesn't warrant the kind of bother it could get me into if I talked about it. Most people don't complain about tactile hallucinations, but hearing things, often derogatory, is different. One of the young girls from Mabledon has auditory hallucinations that she cannot cope with. Her father also has them but he ignores them. He doesn't understand what her problem is, and she has no idea how he can dismiss it.

I tell Stan about the sensual dancing – I'm worried that being three stops short of Plaistow is part and parcel of the job. He laughs, "Come on Sweets – you're as sane as anyone. You got through your teenage years didn't you? You *must* be resilient." He's right, I must be.

—∿—

Selina is a new admission. She is as *mad as a meat cleaver*, – one of Sister's quaint phrases. At first glance you would say Female Admission is *plush* with its rich velvet curtains (puce, which sounds disgusting), though they suit the building. But for all the richness, there aren't any private rooms, only two dormitories. They're even less private than Male Admission because the corridor walls don't go up to the ceiling. On the plus side the northern light from the massive windows floods through the dormitories and onto the carpeted hallway and the polished wooden floor of the dayroom. On the downside, any wailing reaches the ears of everyone.

Sister tries to organise a bed dance and surround Selina by ladies least likely to thump her. She isn't a danger to herself or anyone else so she doesn't warrant isolation in one of the secure rooms, but she *will* annoy some of the other patients, possibly most of them. She is a South African half-caste, with one white parent and one African parent. I confess, to my

39

shame, that I don't see a problem here. In Britain having skin the colour of coffee is hardly unusual and as soon as everyone ends up some shade of latte the better as far as I can see. I am not advocating ditching your culture, a bit jealous really because as a displaced person (in my eyes), I don't feel as if I have any culture. My upbringing wasn't hung up on skin colour. I am aware not everyone shares my take on life – racial hatred is a real and horrible thing even in 1980s England. The outlook in South Africa is very different.

I am given a quick lesson in apartheid. Being half white in South Africa means Selina is simply *not allowed*. Her parents have broken the law. You can be what is described as *coloured* – which means one parent is Indian or some other non-white of foreign origin – or white if you are Japanese! The Chinese have been excluded from immigration since 1904, but any descendants of those long-ago immigrants to South Africa are considered coloured except in some areas where they are black. You can be a black African, and there are a lot of different options there divided by many languages although I probably wouldn't be able to tell the difference visually. Or you can be white, as in European mainly. It is illegal for a white person to have sex with an African (black) or coloured person, so to have a half-white child is impossible without two people having broken the Immorality Act of 1927. White people can't marry anyone other than other whites either because of the 1949 Prohibition of Mixed Marriages Act.

The more I learn the more I realise apartheid is an affront to humanity. How come I don't know all this? It takes me a while for the ramifications to sink in. Either she is the result of a rape – illegal on several levels – or her parents will have been put in jail (originally up to four years for a black woman and up to five years for a white man, and in 1957 the terms of imprisonment were increased to seven years each). I think Selina will have been born before then. I guess she could have been kept secret and her parents never seen with her, but it sounds difficult to organise. Or she was dumped. My head is spinning. Sister assures me she needs two bouts of ECT and will be on her way. She has taken two weeks' annual leave from her job at the bank and everything will be quickly sorted. I am doubtful because she seems very mad to me! She is talking to people that aren't there, and dancing and twirling, she seems oblivious to the rest of the world, and she can't sit still long enough to eat. Sister assures me she comes in every couple of years and her recovery is astonishing.

But there is a problem. Doctor P, the only fully qualified psychiatrist, has other ideas. He is great – he has some progressive views on treatment, and although he too appears quite crazy (he has a cloak and a spinning green bow tie), he is against needlessly drugging new admissions. He is on a crusade to reduce medication levels (and thus costs) throughout the hospital. He also wants ECT stopped completely. Anyone admitted to Female Admission complaining of depression is prescribed two weeks of twice daily trim trail activity, a decent diet, and occupational therapy in the conservatory.

Someone must accompany new patients around the parklike grounds. There are various strengthening activities dotted along a circular pathway of about two miles and patients are encouraged to build to a jog between the stations. Everyone is happy that I volunteer, and I have never been this fit. Almost everyone improves, even over as short a time as two weeks.

Except Selina. Sister can't get an agreement for ECT, and the weeks are dragging by. Selina should be back at the bank, but she is still floridly psychotic. The prescribed medication has had no effect whatsoever. After six weeks the bank loses patience, they sack her, and she can't pay her rent. Dr P relents – scared, I suspect, of both Ward Sisters who have ganged up on him and become what I can only describe as stroppy. Selina has two rounds of ECT, quickly improves and is discharged to a halfway house. The Sisters are ropable, the psychiatrist has learned to listen to experience and so have I. Selena is jobless and homeless. Apparently, this is progress.

Our initial visit to the ECT suite made me think it was barbaric. The treatment had been mainstream but has become controversial. Inducing seizures isn't new – remember the last insulin therapy us newbies witnessed? And I doubt very much that what we witnessed *was* the last in the world. Seizures have also been induced using drugs, initially camphor, then later pentylenetetrazol (cardiozol) in high doses. Cardiozol is a respiratory stimulant, but its effects can be erratic.

Electricity was deemed safer and more controllable. Initially, patients were simply held down and shocked, but the seizures could be violent. One patient, a Mr Bolam, complained in court about his treatment which resulted in broken bones. Although he didn't win, it did change the way treatment was given. This has become known as the "Bolam Test". In those days it was thought better not to inform patients of potential problems and Mr Bolam complained that although he *had* consented to ECT (he was a patient at the Friern Hospital in 1957), he had not been sedated, held down, nor informed of the possibility of ending up with his bones in bits.

These days patients are given a muscle relaxant (succinylcholine) to stop the flailing about. All you see is a twitch of the toes, but because succinylcholine makes you feel as though you are suffocating since it paralyses your breathing, a short-acting anaesthetic is also given.

I attend the ECT sessions with Selina. There is nothing to see – it barely registers there even *was* a current – she woke up, had a cup of tea, and carried on as if nothing had happened. Not everyone fares as well as her though; headaches and memory loss are common complaints. Some staff have suggested her problems are hysterical because ECT is usually a course of at least six treatments. Two treatments are not supposed to fix anything. In my opinion her problems have nothing to do with hysteria – no one loses their job and their home through wanting two ECTs and *playing up* to get them!

There *is* someone here who is hysterical, though, and she also has epilepsy. She appears to have schizophrenia, but no one will diagnose it. Not because it is supposed to be precluded by epilepsy (even though that isn't true), but because she appears to be pretending. She is fine when she thinks no one is watching, but at other times she responds to what she says are voices, she looks wildly around and wails or stands about in a trance. She claims to be seriously ill. Selina was crazy all the time. Sister has had enough. She tries to get rid of the patient by suggesting she should go to the conservatory and find something useful to do, but the girl won't go, claiming to be far too ill. Sister hatches a plan and sends me to the pharmacy for a sugar pill.

When I return with the pill Sister makes quite the performance, telling the patient it is considered a dangerous drug, only to be given in extreme circumstances. "It can cause a blood pressure drop – you could pass out."

I am concerned the theatrics might make the patient smell a rat. Then I get it: Sister is looking to have consent from the patient, and I am the witness.

Sister continues, "Are you sure you want to take this pill? Would you prefer seeing how things are at occupational therapy?"

The patient's response is clear. She is *so* ill. There *is* something not right about this girl. Wanting to be in hospital isn't normal, her epilepsy is well-controlled. At this point the theatrics are with the patient – she desperately *needs* the drug. Sister hands it to her with a big glass of water, she swallows it and immediately passes out. We carry her to the dormitory and the ward is peaceful for the rest of the day.

Sister is in so much trouble! One of the junior doctors has squealed to Dr P. The translation for placebo from Latin is, *I will please.* Using a treatment that makes no difference, or *should* make no difference, has been in use for at least two hundred years. Sister is in trouble because it is deceptive. Of course if a psychiatrist had prescribed it, then it would have been OK. I am astonished it worked so well. I believe there is something going on that we don't understand.

I am almost at the end of my stint, and I have learned more here than anywhere, I'm so grateful for the care and support I have been given. The Irish girl has been shipped back to Ireland; it is a wake-up call. There isn't an us and them – it could be anyone, and not a lot of people know that.

Honda 400 Four (CB400F)

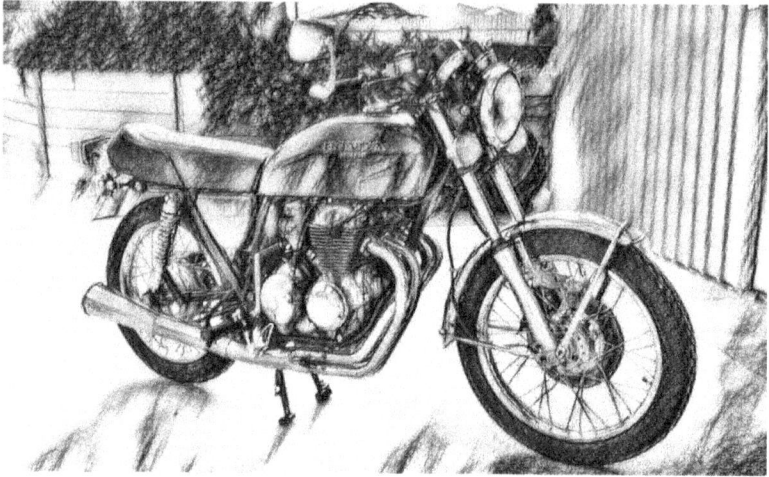

Personal photograph reimagined by lunapic.com

Chapter 6: Sitting Ducks

Squashing into the never-worn uniform provided back in January makes me realise I should eat less. I confess to baking a cake each week. I cover it in clotted cream and roll it in nuts. There are only the two of us to eat it and we should stop.

Female Hospital is the last placement of the year. At this end of the hospital the magnificent building deteriorates. Literally, there is no one left to care, by now most of the patients have either outlived their relatives or been abandoned and it looks like building maintenance has given up as well. Back in the day it is unlikely anyone lived long enough to get this far. The male and female hospital units were only added because patients are living longer. The faded yellow paint is peeling, the lino in the dormitory is cracked, and damp patches show in the lounge carpet. Unlike the ornate ceilings resplendent in the rest of the building here we have asbestos tiles. They look like they will fall at any minute. Some of these patients will have been admitted as youngsters to the grandeur of Female Admission in the East Wing. They will have danced in the ballroom at night and worked in the gardens or the crystal conservatory by day. Gradually working their way west. Female Long Stay, Female Geriatrics, Female Hospital – the next step is the chapel.

The old dears are barely mobile. The enrolled nurse, who seems to do all the work, tells me almost all of them have had either a hip replacement or a fractured pelvis. She whips back a sheet to display surgical scars. Most of these ducks are incontinent. Probably secondary to poor mobility. Consequently, the place smells. There is one dormitory with thirty beds and no privacy. The hospital is not big on privacy at either end, the prospects of a single room are better in the middle. Each bed has one small wooden cupboard on wheels, topped with a thin drawer, there is barely enough space to get the patients in and out of bed.

Most are on weight loss diets and being treated for depression. I can understand why they are depressed, but most

45

of them are tiny and the only reason they might weigh any less is because there are two lifting machines, thirty patients, and one machine is not working. The staff are as old and frail as the lifting devices.

In the 1940s hips were not replaced when destroyed by arthritis or (commonly) tuberculosis; instead the femoral head would be cut off. It isn't that there weren't alternatives, but there wasn't any standard of care so simplicity ruled. In fact, a guy named Sir Robert Jones would put gold foil over the femoral head as a means of alleviating pain; other ideas were to cover the head with pig's bladder, but often stability or mobility would be compromised. Informed consent wasn't a thing, so surgeons could do what they liked. In 1923 some replacement hip joints were made from glass, which seemed OK initially, but then they began to shatter so Bakelite (an early plastic) and Pyrex were tried. Eventually vitallium (an amalgam of cobalt, chromium and molybdenum that was already in use in dentistry) was used in 1937. Then came custom-made stainless-steel implants fixed with screws and bolts, but these loosened easily. In the 1960s a polytetrafluoroethylene (PTFE) cup was used by Sir John Charnley, but they also wore down and resulted in inflammatory reactions.

Charnley tried a lot of different techniques but most of the patients in Female Hospital will have either PTFE cups or replacement femoral heads combined with cups of alternate materials put in place using cement. Most of the replacement joints did not last well and had to be removed.

This may not be the sole reason for their poor condition though, because anaesthetic in the older patient doesn't have a great outcome either, frequently being followed by cognitive decline. It makes me determined that should Stan need a hip replacement he will have an epidural. I read about this very recently – epidurals have been available for labour for a while and have been used with good effect for a hip replacement just this year (Hole et al, 1980).

—∿—

Iraq has invaded Iran. You might think this is half a world away and not very relevant, but we have two junior doctors here, good friends until today. Now things are frosty. The Iraqi guy is small – my guess would be about 5 ft 6 inches tall – and prematurely balding, The Iranian guy tells everyone he is 6 ft 12 inches, and certainly my eye level is equal to his crotch. He isn't a beanpole; his girth is reasonable for someone of his height. He's simply a giant person. Both are friendly guys. I can't imagine they could fight each other – the little guy would get squished! You would think they had each kidnapped the other's mother and raped their sisters the way they have torn each other apart this afternoon. The tension isn't helped by the six o'clock news showing graphic images of bombs being dropped.

Because these two come as a pair and work across the whole hospital, the icy tentacles of their current relationship will drop the temperature everywhere! Doctor P isn't interested in their sudden animosity. I think he is from Sri Lanka. Medication was supposed to be the answer to everything, but it has come at significant cost. Not only a budget blowout, but the side effects in some cases are worse than the original complaint. He has slashed the antidepressants for these elderly ladies. He wants to see if any of them really are depressed or if the medication is contributing to their confusion. He also wants them weighed.

I am hoping to learn about caring for patients because I go to my medical secondment in the new year, and so far no one has really needed any physical care. I have learned to make a bed with hospital corners, which hardly any of the patients appreciate. They make their own beds for the most part; I help on occasion, and critique if called upon. I hate hospital corners too – the first thing I do with a made bed I plan to sleep in is mess it up. I can't sleep with tucked in sheets. I have taken blood pressure and pulse, mostly for practice. I haven't bathed anyone, or even given them a wash. I have played a *lot* of badminton and board games, gone for walks, and made good use of the trim trail. I have taken people to appointments, helped them fill out bewildering paperwork and assisted with medication rounds, but actual physical care? Not so much. I won't be able to wriggle out of washing and bed making here.

We start weighing tomorrow; it won't be as easy as it sounds because half of the patients can't stand. I also am not sure how you would know if they were depressed because half of them don't talk either.

The dinner trolley comes, and I start sorting out the meals; some of the plastic lids have roughly scrawled labels; diabetic, low residue or MAOI. This last one is a special diet for patients prescribed antidepressants called monoamine oxidase inhibitors. These have various sorts of brand names (Nardil, Marplan, Parnate) but they all require a diet low in tyramine. Tyramine is an amino acid naturally found in the body that helps regulate blood pressure amongst other things, and the MAOI drugs block its breakdown. The thing is that you get tyramine in the protein in your diet, and if too much builds up where the antidepressant is blocking its breakdown, it can result in a serious (deadly) rise in blood pressure.

Tyramine is especially high in things like cheese and cured or smoked meats but also in foods you might not think of such as sauces, pickled foods, beer, sherry, snow peas, broad beans and even bananas. I did query the banana thing, and it is limited to banana skins. I don't know anyone who eats banana skin, but the dietician did tell me that the little stringy bits along the ridges of a ripe banana can also be high in tyramine and are hard to remove. I am fairly concerned that suddenly stopping the antidepressant medication these frail old ladies have been on for many years, might cause problems with withdrawal. I am told it doesn't happen, but there will still be residual medication in their circulation.

The Ward Sister interferes with the meals, telling me that only the diabetic patients need the right meal – she can see there aren't any overweight patients. It's a bit late to hope they gain anything before we weigh them.

"Just give them out!" she bellows.

I stand my ground over the MAOI meals. Sister goes ballistic, summons me to her office and slams the door. She is reporting me for insubordination. She is on the verge of screaming at me. I am to go home immediately. She will not be having me back.

Oh shit, the last thing I need is trouble. I don't even know what I have done – all I said was the MAOI meals need to be continued for fourteen days. I know this. We went over it in school when the dietician came to lecture us. I have also read about it in MIMs; this isn't secret stuff, and she should know. I *had* to say something because these old ladies could die.

—∿—

Stan isn't even there; I am greeted by our insane cat. The next day I am summoned to the nursing school to explain.

I have been rehearsing my defence all night, but they disarm me right away – they totally know why I did what I did and agree Sister should know better. Her grievance is that I said it in front of everyone. Which is true. They point out that if I want to be a registered nurse then there will be occasions when I will need to tell someone their work is less than optimal. I protest that she had argued with me, loudly, though I initially made mention quietly. She could easily have said, "Oh yes, go ahead." But she argued that I was wrong, so my back was in a corner. My tutors say I should have asked to talk to her. But I was worried the enrolled nurses would have handed the meals out willy nilly while I reasoned with her in the privacy of her office. I am not convinced she would have backed down even then. I feel the only reason she has is because she's had time to check things out. Apparently she will let me back if I apologise.

I apologise, but the frosty reception I get deteriorates after dinner (where everyone gets their designated meal). As a student it is my job, along with the enrolled nurse, to get the clothes ready for the morning. We choose matching dresses and cardigans – hopefully they also belong to the patient so we know they will fit, but they go to the laundry in bags and come back mixed up. We don't have unlimited time for this job

49

because we also need to get everyone into bed. Most of them are wet so they need a decent wash.

For two people to get thirty mostly immobile people washed and into bed is hard work. We use the functioning lifting machine for the heavier patients but some we have to carry. We try to help one another. A lot of the ladies are clearly underweight – and we have proof they are because we spent all afternoon weighing them. Some of them are under forty kg. I had to translate the weight for everyone. Most of them are between five and six stone, and some even less; no one needs to diet. They probably haven't for a very long time, if they ever did.

The thing is, as we put them to bed I notice that the clothes I had carefully hung on the hangers for the morning shift are different. Initially I don't properly notice, then I think something is off, then I am sure these are not the clothes I hung out. I don't say anything but the next day I take careful note of the clothes I choose. Sure enough, as we put the old dollies to bed the clothes have all changed.

I mention it to my colleague. I thought she was joking when she suggested Sister was changing them. Surely not? But she is. Every evening shift, whatever clothes I get ready she changes. I can't not bother to do the job; I am not looking for a fight. She simply has the pip with me and so both our times are wasted when we could be doing something more constructive.

Like I learned from Female Admission – it isn't us and them; sometimes the lunatics are running the asylum.

There is another disturbing aspect to Female Hospital, apart from the ignorant and nutty Ward Sister and underweight patients. The old ladies are now throwing up. I am certain it has to do with the sudden cessation of antidepressants. But what do I know? I also have a problem with the Buxton chairs. The patients spend their entire day in these chairs. These are the kind that are thrown backwards whether the patient wants to be lying back staring at the ceiling or not. It hardly seems worth having a TV since no one can see it. Some of the staff are very adept at the throwback and the chairs thud as they are slung back at speed. I can see the old ladies' spindly necks snapping.

Not that they're all old – there is one woman here who is twenty-nine. Her children are nine and ten, but she doesn't recognise them. She *is* mobile – or would be if she weren't tied to her chair and slung back like everyone else. She has already broken her ankle going over the wall. I don't blame her; I would risk it too. She has early onset Alzheimer's. Twenty-nine is at the extreme end of the age range even for early onset dementia and it is terribly sad. She wants to run away; her husband and children visit but she doesn't know who they are, and they leave in tears. I leave in tears because I don't have any power to change her situation.

The other thing that bothers me a lot is the fact that no one thinks to put glasses on the patients. I see them in their empty top drawers, covered in dust. Without my glasses, not only can I not see, but I can't hear either. I put my glasses on to answer the phone and I am not alone in that! We rely on people's faces much more than we think, though that doesn't really account for the phone thing. Commonly there are hearing aids and false teeth in the drawers too, also covered in dust. This results in a problem when a rare relative turns up and we find essential dentures or expensive hearing aids have gone missing and the staff can't recall the last time they saw them.

I am glad this rotation is over. I thought it would prepare me for the medical ward in the new year. Hopefully that won't be like this, and the Ward Sister will be more welcoming.

Back in school I struggle to be in class when I know there is a spot waiting for me in front of the fire in the library. We have a test to see if we are worthy of another year of slave labour – and it transpires we are. It's already dark during the final ride of the year along the sweeping driveway exiting the grounds of Darenth Park. I ride carefully to avoid the piles of slippery leaves, yet still my Honda slides out from under me. I am not hurt. The bike doesn't even look damaged, but something is wrong. When I gather my balls to get back on it, I find the gears won't change.

It's a long way home in one gear. When Stan takes it apart he can see that the gears are too close together. The Honda 400 Four has four inline cylinders and six gears. Six gears are unnecessary on a motorbike. Inevitably they are too close together. Now they are also worn. They wobble and catch on one another. It will have momentarily seized the back wheel which will have locked up, resulting in being dumped in the gutter. He quickly puts it back together.

"We need to unload this Sweets. It's downright dangerous." We swap it for a car, a dark blue 1970 Triumph 1500 cc, front-wheel drive. Neither of us has a licence to drive the thing.

Chapter 7: Failure is Not an Option

Wearing a uniform, even though the dress is impractically tight around the thighs for the job, is OK. I love the snuggly cloak although I rarely wear it because it could be a danger on a motorbike. The mustard colour of my second-year belt is awful and betrays my status to those in the know. But the simplicity of it appeals to me. It has a niftily designed interlocking clasp; you could put it on one-handed with some practice. Plus, the slightly elasticated webbing is handy for those bloated days.

I don't know what to expect; this is proper nursing at Joyce Green Hospital – a general hospital – and on a medical ward. This is precisely what I said I wouldn't do. Walking through the green swing doors, I am hit with the unfamiliar smell of disinfectant. The lino is obviously enthusiastically polished and lacks the cracks I have come to expect. I'm not going to have it in my house. We put carpet in the kitchen. Completely impractical but so cheap we can swap it out when it gets too bad. The Female Medical ward is huge and light. It has high pointed ceilings rather than the flat ornate ones of Stone House. Privacy is marginally better because the beds have curtains around each one. Flimsy and a bit tatty, but something at least. The problem with the mustard belt is that patients aware of the system think I am a second-year nurse. They don't know that on a general medical ward I am a complete beginner.

Sister greets me: "Get out of my sight. I hate psych nurses – they are a complete waste of time. If you must be here, you will keep out of my way."

It isn't the welcome I anticipated. There are three other student nurses starting today. Two first years and a third year. They are general nurses; Sister doesn't mind them. I'm the only waste of space. Of course I'm quite used to it from school.

She lists the things she expects me to do: make beds and bath people – in bed! On Female Hospital we bathed the old ladies in a bath. We did wash their nether regions in bed if they

53

were wet – essential to prevent them getting sore. We shoved a rubber mackintosh under their bums and did the essential bits, not a whole bath. Sister makes it clear that I am not welcome to watch any procedure unless I do it in my own time and ensure I keep out of her way. The other students are as shocked as I am.

I spend the first day familiarising myself with the ward, reading stuff, talking to patients, and feeling as if I have been hit around the head with a cricket bat because I'm not sure what to do. On the way home I call in at the nursing school. They know there have been some difficulties but say I should simply make the best of it. None of this seems right to me. Joyce Green is supposed to be a teaching hospital.

The following day the alternate Ward Sister is on duty, and she apologises. It seems the older and more senior Ward Sister's mother has been incarcerated in Stone House. She built, and lit, a fire in the lounge (which doesn't have a fireplace). Apparently I am to blame! Of course I'm not. I don't even know who this woman is, but lighting fires is taken seriously. The Senior Sister thinks it is a conspiracy and blames anyone associated with psychiatry. Privately I think she has some marbles on the loose as well. However, I increase my status quickly with the younger Sister as she quizzes us students about the concentration of salt in a saline drip. Since I'm a psych nurse Sister doesn't expect me to know this. Truly this was on M.A.S.H. last night (season 8 episode 9)! The only decent TV show to come out of the United States and not one of the general students watched it, or if they did then they weren't paying attention. I give it a decent amount of time (OK, a minimal amount of time) for the general students to show off – before I do.

So, day two and I'm dancing!

This is very different from what I'm used to. I have made beds, even with hospital corners, but usually I help a patient make their bed and I can accept a bit of a mess. Here they are inspected. Some of the patients are still in bed and an elaborate system of rolling them about is expected to produce a pristine bed with hospital corners and zero creases. Please spare me from ever ending up in one.

Then a woman takes the biscuit. She is calling, her voice frail. She is young and fit and has chest pain, but no one is thinking very much of it. Query wind is what it says in her notes. Still, she is in hospital, and I'm supposed to be nice. I ask her what I can do for her.

"Nurse, nurse, pass my tissues."

As close as can be to her right arm, which is not broken and does not have a drip in it, is a box of tissues. I bite my lip hard and pass the tissues, moving away without a word, lest it be scathing. Although the proposed emptying of the loony bins has barely happened, it has been drilled into us in our classes what a problem institutionalisation is and how it can start in small ways. Nan told me about some of her old chums being released. I didn't know you could know so many mad people but oh dear, this permanent incarceration is so much worse.

Nan died, her passing unexpected. She was blown over by the wind that swirled around the high-rise she lived in. Whenever we visited we would hold hands, my brother and I between our parents, to get from the car to the entrance of the tower block without being blown away. The coroner said she had a heart attack because she was blown over; she didn't fall because of the heart attack. I'm not sure how you can tell but that was the story.

Before she died I can remember her becoming distressed after visiting an old friend she hadn't seen for fifty years. The way she explained it was characteristic of her generation. Her friend had got herself into trouble. This makes it sound as if only one person is involved in this version of trouble when we all know it takes two. Back in the day when children (they were children) became pregnant they disappeared. Pregnancy out of wedlock was supposed to be rare. Girls would have a speedy wedding since marriageable age for girls up until 1929 was twelve. If the male in question had scarpered, then the chances were that the girl would end up in the workhouse. There would be no way Nan could have stayed in touch, and by the middle of the century these girls would likely to have been moved to the County Lunatic Asylum as the workhouses were closed. The asylums were deliberately out of area, a geographic cure for an embarrassing problem.

With the push to close the asylums, women who were pregnant on entry but not insane (though that probably changed) were some of the first to be shifted out. They had already paid the price with the loss of their child and any future family. They likely ended their pregnancy working in a laundry, often run by nuns. Shifting to the lunatic asylum may have been optional, but if it was it would have been Hobson's choice. In 1929, long after Nan's friends had disappeared, the running of the workhouses was transferred to the county councils. To be fair they had become refuges of the sick and disabled because anyone able-bodied tried to stay well away. By 1948 the National Health Service had taken over any workhouses that hadn't closed. Nan was upset because her friend, now discharged from the asylum, was a wreck. She had been moved into a flat with three other elderly ladies. They couldn't cook, shop, manage money or catch a bus. More progress.

Glancing back at the woman with the tissue box problem, she appears so helpless. Am I helping her? I don't think so. It might be a small thing, but learned helplessness is the start of a slippery slope.

The Senior Ward Sister is as good as her word. I watch a bone marrow aspiration taken from the sternum after my shift has finished. One of the first-year nurses is there too, during work time – she needs the experience and I do not. She doesn't get the experience because she passes out. I grip the bed so I don't follow her. I hear the bone cracking as the large needle is screwed in. A later lumbar puncture isn't any better. I am trying to learn, but what with missing meals and staying late I'm finding it hard to put heart and soul into this.

—∿—

The morning of the 27 April 1981 I wake up to a whiteout. The severe snowstorms that have crossed the country the past few days have finally hit Kent. I couldn't see how I would get to work. Not by motorbike, anyway. After swapping the dodgy Honda for a car (though I don't know if we won out of the deal) my bike licence doubles as a learner licence for a car, but I am supposed to have a qualified driver with me. I have been using Stan's little Yamaha trail bike to get to work but it's impossible in these conditions, so I'll have to risk the car. I can't see the police chasing me down on a day like today. It looks terrifying out there.

In fact, the roads are deserted. This is usually a journey of about thirty-five minutes, sometimes more. Today it is a lot more and I'm late, but instead of getting told off – the night shift who are still there because NO ONE has turned-up – welcome me with open arms. It takes a few minutes for the whole scenario to seep into my challenged brain. The journey has taken every bit of wit and now, keen to escape, the night staff think I am taking over. After all I'm a second-year student – see my smart mustard belt? Failing to get my point across, I watch them flee, and I'm left amongst seriously endangered patients. They don't realise their greatest danger is me. I have no idea what I'm doing – after all, I don't need to know anything!

I call the hospital Matron; she tells me to take charge and do the best I can not to kill anyone. Right. I phone the nursing school – this is surely wrong? They tell me to do whatever I am told. Some people live close enough to walk. What the hell is wrong with them? Anyone who has a heart attack today will die. I'm not sure if I should bath them or corral all the beds so I can see everyone at the same time and simply watch them. They can stay dirty.

The breakfast trolley arrives in time to save me from a complete nervous breakdown. Breakfast is within my skill set. The drug round is not! To dish out medication I need to have passed my drugs assessment which is a year two assessment, and I haven't done it. I wouldn't be doing it here anyway because I need to demonstrate my ability with modern psychiatric medication which is being churned out at an alarming rate. I phone Matron again. She can't have me killing people by dishing out lollies to the wrong person so she will come and at least do that.

Matron hands out the pills and finds one hospital aide to help. They know more than I do but are equally terrified about the responsibility. It is better having another body here though, and most of the patients are keen to do whatever they can to make our lives better. Unfortunately, it is the more seriously ill people who want to help and that only adds to the stress.

This is the longest day of my short life. On the way home I skid to avoid an oncoming car as it slides onto my side of the road. I am so scared. It occurs to me that since I'm driving without supervision I have probably voided my insurance as well. Plus, I'm an inexperienced driver. I hate this placement, and I hate the lazy, good-for-nothing staff who couldn't be bothered to even walk to get there. Lucky no one is dead.

$$-\sqrt{\sqrt{}}-$$

Weeks ago I applied to a temp agency, hoping to pick up some holiday work as a nursing assistant. I'd thought I would have some kind of competency by now. I have two weeks back at school, then I have been booked to work at the Medway Hospital aged care unit in the half-term break. I should cope with oldies.

It turns out they are as barmy as everywhere else I've been. One of the staff wants me gone because she is having menopausal issues, and when she finds I am a trainee psych nurse she thinks I will dob her into the authorities and she'll lose her job. I can't win. The agency redirects me to the diabetic ward. I understand the biology, but nothing at all about the care.

It is quite illuminating. Mostly these are children and teenagers. They don't need much care, which is just as well. I do a lot of pee testing. I can detect ketones in urine without using the test strips. There is a smell to it, and it's also on their breath. Pear drops. I use the sticks for evidence. Even with my superpowers I can't tell how high the levels are, and too high can be fatal.

Ketones find their way into the urine when the body is burning fat for fuel. It will do this when there is insufficient glucose for the cells to use for energy. In diabetes this can be because there is insufficient insulin to allow glucose from the diet to be taken into the cell to be used for fuel. It could be the person hasn't eaten enough or has used up glucose by exercising more than usual. Or a combination of all of these things. One of the medical students on her psych placement on Female Admission was diabetic and always had two gingernut biscuits in her pocket – emergency supplies in case she was on her feet longer than expected or for some reason morning tea got delayed. She was clued up and fit and healthy. The Medway patients are either too young to be so responsible or have recently been diagnosed and need to learn how to control their blood glucose levels. Some youngsters have hopeless parents. Some are also what is known as fragile – their diabetes has been difficult to bring under any kind of control. Diabetics are prone to infections – cuts struggle to heal – and some patients are quite sick, but I don't hang out with those very sick children.

In the 1700s (the age of enlightenment, apparently) doctors used to taste the urine. In India they were smart enough to use ants to see if they were attracted by the sugar. I can smell sugar as well as ketones. I don't take sugar in my tea, but I can smell if one grain has managed to get in it – say if someone has used an unwashed teaspoon to stir my tea. Juvenile diabetes has been on the rise. It used to be considered very rare, and before the advent of insulin in the 1920s children generally died quite quickly even when they were treated with diets extra low in carbohydrate. A recent study (most of the work has been done in Denmark) has shown an upwards creep in the number of young children being diagnosed over the last few years but no one seems to know why. Several of the parents tell me there was nothing wrong with their child until they had tonsillitis or some other childhood virus and then they went downhill. It has been shown their pancreas isn't producing enough insulin. The treatment is insulin by injection.

We have learned in class that there are other types of diabetes, like diabetes insipidus, which isn't the same thing at all. I remember it makes you pee a lot, but it doesn't have to do with uncontrolled glucose levels and is very rare. We also briefly learned about diabetes mellitus (mellitus means honey) which has become known as type two diabetes to differentiate it from juvenile diabetes. Sometimes it is called late-onset diabetes because it affects adults rather than children. This does lead to high glucose levels in the blood, but I have never seen anyone with it. The body makes enough insulin but the cells ignore it so the glucose still doesn't get into the cells where it can be used for energy. I have no idea how you might treat it because giving insulin for the cell to ignore seems pointless. There is also a type of diabetes you can get when you are pregnant. I don't know anything about that either, but it must be more common because I have at least heard of it. I already knew of two people with juvenile diabetes treated by insulin injections and now I'm in an entire ward of them, so it must be the most common.

There is a conundrum – the old ducks in Female Hospital whose dinners came with diabetic scrawled on the plastic lids could not have had juvenile diabetes. It would have been a killer when they were children. You *can* get it as an adult, usually following an infection, but it's rare. I hadn't thought about it at the time. Thinking wasn't encouraged, and after my run in with Sister I kept my head down.

At least here I am learning something useful, and I'm being paid a decent enough wage – especially since this is on top of my minimum training wage!

I have been doing something useful for Stan as well, I see him so cold getting off his motorbike that his knees are stiff, so I have knitted him a jumper. I'm not known for these homely skills – it is a complex pattern with cables, a diamond front panel and the rest looks like basket weave. He is thrilled with it, he hasn't taken it off since I finished it.

Chapter 8: Care in the Community

Time spent in the school has been more interesting than usual, plus the library fire is out – much too early in my opinion. It means I'm more inclined to pay attention to things other than my growing collection of case-notes.

We had a guest speaker, an environmental health officer. This is quite interesting to me because I have toyed with the idea of training for this in the past, but given my few qualifications didn't think I had much chance. I am fascinated to discover there is more to it than retrieving restaurant rats. The biggest thing that sticks in my mind is the family who complained they were struggling to get in and out of their house. When the officer got there he found a full-blown tree had grown through the concrete step. The front door could barely open. It had become more and more difficult to get in and out over the years and it blows my mind that the family had not thought to do something before reaching this point.

It makes me think about fat people. People are getting bigger. Some are confined to bed. A woman was admitted to the medical unit at Joyce Green who arrived on the floor of the ambulance because she couldn't fit on the patient trolley. Before we know it, people will be stuck in their homes not because of a tree growing through the doorstep but because they can't fit through the door. At what point would you notice that the door is getting suspiciously narrow?

—∿—

The environmental health stuff is still on my mind; after all I'm only training as a nurse because I couldn't find anything else. I was hopelessly out of my depth on the medical ward. It still astonishes me no one died, but I am feeling more confident about community nursing. We have each been assigned to a General Practitioner clinic. The clinic itself is a soulless 70s-designed building. It is modern and clean but doesn't have any architectural merit – fit for purpose, nothing more.

Feeling a bit self-conscious. I pile my crash helmet, boots and coat in a corner. I'm having driving lessons, but I failed my first test so am still on the trail bike. I suppose there's nothing wrong with that, though a woman has already had a go at me for riding it in the woods. She wasn't happy about the zing, zing noise it makes. It doesn't do anything for my street credibility out on the road either.

The welcome couldn't be better. They laid on morning tea to introduce me to the entire team. I'm going to be happy here, I know it. Valerie (not Val) is the Health Visitor. She is going to take me under her wing. I will also spend time with the Midwife, the District Nurse and one of the General Practitioners. I'm invited to the staff meetings, and in a few weeks the sales rep for a drug company will put on an afternoon tea. I was taught never to turn down free food.

After morning tea Valerie takes me to a community care house for the mentally ill. These types of places are springing up with the expectation that they will take the people emptied from the bins as well as new patients. The point is to prevent people from ever entering a lunatic asylum. The very sick will go to specialised units within a general hospital; Oonagh, went to the one in Joyce Green. I'm hoping to get a stint there at some stage. Margaret Thatcher, Prime Minister – and lunatic if ever I saw one – is still intent on emptying the bins though I don't see much progress. She has done some good for the nation (the rate of inflation is down) although now unemployment is rising.

A Government paper proposed abolition of the asylums for the mentally handicapped in 1971, and Darenth Park was listed for closure in 1973, yet I don't see anything happening. In 1975 the government decided the entire mental health system would be disbanded and local councils would be responsible for the mental wellbeing of their own community.

The community care home that Valerie has brought me to is one destined to replace the bins but can only take a handful of patients. They aim that no one will stay for long, with a two-year maximum. The set-up is quite interesting. The purpose-built brick house has two floors and mostly single rooms. The staff have been chosen specifically for their personalities. They are looking to employ a gay male nurse but are not allowed to advertise explicitly. They are after marketing ideas. I know exactly the person they need but he wouldn't come and work for them (and denies being gay) because he has a lucrative number taking old institutionalised rich men on holiday. I mean nothing dodgy by this – the wealthy families are happy with the arrangement, it makes them feel good, and I would trust him with my life.

It isn't surprising gay men aren't rushing to announce themselves. In England homosexuality was punishable by death until 1861 – the last couple being executed in 1835 – and homosexuality was decriminalised under the Sexual Offences Act of 1967 but this was only in a limited number of circumstances. The restrictions that came with this "progressive" law means men are still effectively locked in the closet. For instance, to have male-to-male sex, three conditions must be satisfied; it has to be consensual (I should hope so!), the participants must be over 21 despite recommendation from the Home Office that it be reduced to 18 (it's 16 for heterosexuality), and it can only be between two people in a private space. This is where problems occur because two people is specifically the people involved, and a hotel room is not considered a private space. The two people can be in a private home, but if someone else lives there then it is illegal, even if the extra person isn't in the same room. Things are worse in Scotland where the Criminal Justice Act of 1980 has only just come into force on the 1st of February this year and don't bother to go to Ireland (North or the Republic) at all!

The community home has a bossy, motherly type woman who seems to be ruling the roost but isn't in charge. The guy in charge is rather relaxed – you might even say an introvert. Unusual, but he is amiable and knowledgeable. The idea is the residents will naturally find someone within the staff they can relate to. They haven't been open long enough to see how things work out.

It makes me think about my personality; how would I fit in? I am twenty-one but I have seen more in my life than most people. I have already been burnt, yet I remain mostly cheerful – a glass half full type. I'm certainly not shy although I appreciate my alone time. I have calmed down from the sassy teenager I was when my brains were very nearly fried on amphetamine. I set out to be a drug addict, determined to die before I was thirty-five. Then I changed my mind. I struggle with something, though I'm not sure what. If I'm honest, I'm grateful I am still alive. If I worked here someone would surely relate to me. Presuming I don't turn into an environmental health officer, then this is a possibility.

The 1962 Hospital Plan for England and Wales predicted that half of all mental health beds would be gone by 1975. People would either stay at home or live in community accommodation. Acute-psychiatric units in general hospitals would be the reserve of the seriously disturbed. Where the large numbers of long-stay patients would go is anyone's guess. The community-care place we saw this morning could end up as a dumping ground. Some people think families will take them in, but even from my limited experience I can see families are either overwhelmed or have made it clear by their total lack of involvement that they aren't interested. Joyce Green and other hospital-based units wouldn't be putting up with people staying for ages. This is a long way past 1975, and it still hasn't happened. If the plan is to wait for all the patients in the long-stay wards to die, then many years will pass before those big old Victorian asylums can be torn down. Of course they might fall down first.

I'm shocked at the age of some of the mothers-to-be that I meet when I go out with the midwife. She tells me she doesn't always even get to see the very youngest pregnant children. I know this isn't the wealthiest area, but there is a real sense of lost hope amongst the youth here. Not only here, but there have been riots around the country, notably a few weeks ago in Brixton where operation *Swamp-81* saw 943 people stopped and searched within five days as the use of the *Sus* law is out of hand. "Ghost Town" by The Specials has become a theme song for the unrest. The song talks of fighting on the dance floor.

Some of these young and pregnant girls are thrilled, anticipating a love they have never known. At sixteen I would not have coped. These girls are even younger.

The next day I am out with Valerie again. A day job instead of shift, which makes life simpler. We have two girls to visit this morning, both twelve years old, plus their babies. I am reminded that when Nan was a girl they could be married at twelve. These girls are children, not close to being teenagers and that extends to their bodies and their brains –, did they even *have* a first period?

The first has her baby placed in a cardboard box on top of the television. She explains it is warmer than the rest of the house and the baby can be easily watched. Really her parents are caring for the baby, but they don't seem the full quid either. Valerie gives her some kindly advice – the baby will start to wriggle and fall off the TV at some stage – but I can see this is an uphill battle. I don't think any of them should be caring for a baby.

At the next house Valerie shows me the bunk beds in the young girl's bedroom. She hid the pregnancy; in fact she claims she didn't know she was pregnant. She would have been eleven, so perhaps this is true. I had what I can only describe as an experience, aged eleven. Nothing that could leave me pregnant, but something I could neither deal with nor tell anyone about. One morning this girl had stomach cramp before school. She delivered the baby herself and put it under the bunk bed and left for school. I'm not fully up to date with the way deliveries go, but this sounds incredible. I know there is a placenta to think about. The girl's mother seems a bit more with it than the last one and explains that she heard a cry from the bedroom. She couldn't find anything and eventually looked under the bed, thinking a cat had got trapped there, and saw a baby! She has high hopes for the child. I can't see much hope at all.

We check up on a couple of regular mothers, but the youngsters had to take up the bulk of the day – how can you teach a twelve-year-old how to care for a baby in the usual twenty-minute visit? I see there is paperwork, but I can skip over it and check out the clinic itself; tomorrow I hang out with the practice nurse. The health visitor job could be quite rewarding, but I would have to get through training as a general nurse, and I don't think I could. If it were down to me, I would change the system. I would have one year every wannabe nurse would do, and then two years of specialisation in their chosen field. I think students would have a better grip about what they would be letting themselves in for before they signed themselves up for three years. I would have them do intellectual handicap, mental health, general, midwifery, community – it wouldn't be much time in each, but you could learn bed making on the fly surely? Considering it's mostly slave labour anyway you would find out the worst aspects of the job pretty quickly.

As spring turns to summer – things are getting worse and "Ghost Town" becomes an anthem. Margaret Thatcher thinks the upcoming Royal wedding will galvanise the spirit of the nation. She can't see the reality on the street. Prince Charles should have married the woman he loves when he had the chance. There isn't anything wrong with Lady Diana Spencer, but everyone knows she there to provide an heir. Camilla is now married to someone else after the Windsor family determined she was *unsuitable* – he would have had to remove himself from succession – which would be a disaster. Princess Anne is worth more than the rest of them put together, but she is *not* next in line for the throne. Heaven forbid the monarch should be a strong woman – it is after all – the United *King*dom.

Prince Andrew would be next in line. He might fly a helicopter for the navy, but there is something not right about him. Mum always fantasised that I would marry him, enough in itself to make me queasy – but flouncing around in posh frocks and curtseying. I don't think so. Long live QEII.

I get full-frontal gore with the district nurse. Foot ulcers that won't heal and dressings that need changing complete with pus. She does something called debridement, which I can assure you I am never doing. She also takes me to talk to an ex-mental health patient. The woman had attempted suicide several times and now has breast cancer. It has cheered her up no end. We aren't visiting because of her mental health or her cancer; she needs an injection of cobalamin which is vitamin B_{12}. This is because she has pernicious anaemia which wouldn't have been discovered without the cancer diagnosis. There are a whole lot of symptoms of B_{12} deficiency – physical stuff such as pins and needles, prematurely grey hair, nausea and fatigue, but also depression, psychosis… the list goes on, so no wonder she has cheered up! Let's hope she survives the cancer.

Although the lady we just left is not a vegetarian, a diet free from animals and animal products will be short on B_{12}. Vitamin B_{12}, is water soluble (so you pee it out) and essential, i.e., the body needs it and cannot synthesise its own. Vegans and vegetarians often have injections as supplementation.

Not everyone understands it isn't simply a case of not eating animal products. You must be smarter than average – it takes effort and brain power to get proper nutrition without meat. I tried it as a teenager, but even with Mum's help it was tough, so I quit.

Thomas Addison (of Addison's disease fame) had already described pernicious anaemia in the mid-1800s, but it was untreatable and patients died. It is quite likely that women with hysteria, a complaint of the 1800s, had it. In fact, they could have had a variety of diseases, but then – as now – women's complaints were not taken seriously. It was a superhero of mine, Dorothy Hodgkin, who discovered the structure of cobalamin (B_{12}), and won the Nobel prize for chemistry in 1964. She additionally discovered the structures for insulin and penicillin. I wonder how many people are locked into a diagnosis that precludes them from proper care?

It puts me in mind of a friend of my mother-in-law. She has multiple sclerosis and had back pain for years but because of the multiple sclerosis, she was told it was to be expected and nothing could be done. Eventually she went to see a chiropractor. These are people who call themselves doctors, but the medical world calls them witch doctors. She calls them magicians because with a few cracks, her back pain disappeared.

When I was seven, I overheard a conversation between my parents about a mate of Dad's at Hubinuts (as he called it) where he worked. He got paid by how many cabinets he made, not by how long he worked, I thought it was hugely funny because I knew he'd painted the handles of his tools different colours so he could find them quickly. He is colourblind so I couldn't see how it would work but he reckoned it was useful. Mum doesn't let him choose paint or clothes. Now Dad was telling Mum about his work mate who couldn't earn much because he was too slow, but in his case it was because he had multiple sclerosis.

I asked if a doctor could help the man, and Dad said something that stayed with me my whole life. He said that his workmate needed a biochemist. I didn't say anything at the time, but as soon as I got to the library I looked in the big dictionary. There wasn't anything that sounded like it, so I had to ask. I hate help even now, and especially then – asking for help is a last resort. The librarian showed me to a section I had never seen. She said children weren't allowed in the reference library. As I practically lived in the library, and the librarians knew me well, she let me in. We found the words multiple sclerosis, and biochemist. Tough for a seven-year-old, but I worked it out. A biochemist is a new type of scientist, someone studying biology and chemistry. Dad often surprises me; he can barely read and then he comes up with words like these. I wrote it down; it was the second thing on my list.

be a biochemist

Unfortunately getting thrown out of school at fifteen and failing maths and chemistry O-level with a grade that no one in my school had ever got meant I had failed at the first hurdle.

—⋀—

The sales rep is here today, and the table is heavily laden with food. I think this is the extent of the party, but I am wrong. The GPs themselves get colour TVs, the practice manager an overseas holiday. Most of the staff are given stethoscopes, and even I get a hat and a pen. There are chocolates and flowers everywhere. This is a huge con. A bribe. These are sales reps from drug companies, and they are buying favours with their big budgets. I leave my hat and pen behind.

The next day I try and talk to Valerie about it, but she doesn't see my problem. She says the GPs prescribe the medication the patient needs and what the drug companies spend on their sales pitch has no bearing on the prescribing. She believes it and so do the rest of them. I struggle to see how TVs and holidays wouldn't sway you to prescribe their brand over another. Apparently all the drug reps do it. It cements my belief that they are no different to the street dealers cutting their amphetamine with Johnson's baby powder – I have been on the receiving end of that myself! I am disillusioned.

Figure 3. Darenth Park

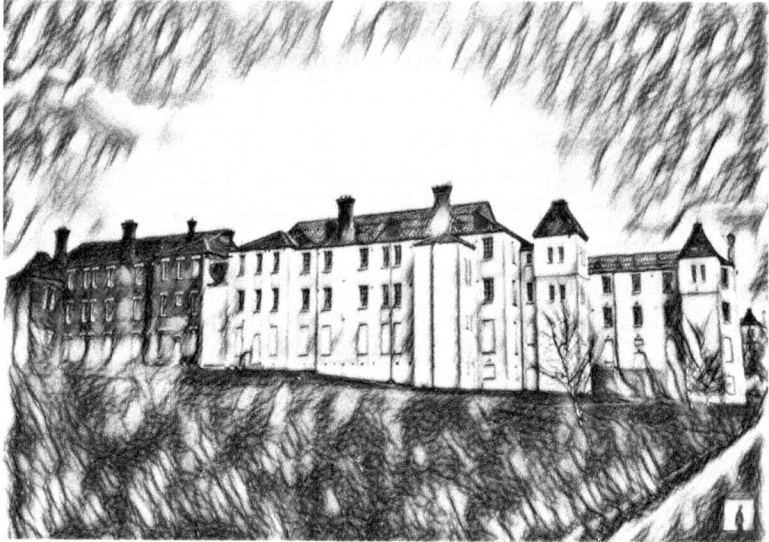

Adapted from "Not-forgotten Asylums in the UK", taken by Jandhands in 1988 after the closure.

Chapter 9: Vera

I trace an upright cross onto the smooth plump buttock with my index finger and stab the needle into the upper outer quadrant. People think student nurses practice their technique by injecting oranges. Not during my training.

"That was nice," she says. "Sorry you are unwell again."

It takes a minute to take in what she has said. We *have* met before – in the first block of my training at Mabledon, the Polish refugee camp. Vera was in the mixed admission ward, an interesting and eclectic assortment of staff and patients. We met on my first day where the staff had made me play in the badminton tournament – all day. Vera didn't play. She was a bit older than the others, unfit and overweight. She seemed happy enough watching her compatriots – mostly young and boisterous. Now it resonates unpleasantly in my mind; despite my uniform, a requirement on long-stay wards, she thinks I am another patient.

I'm eighteen months into my training, so a long time since I first met Vera. I have to get to grips with my first practical assessment – medication. I don't progress unless I pass the practical and this is my first injection. How many first timers have practised on Vera? She has an injection every two weeks to control schizophrenia. Keen to be as informed as possible, I have read her file. Suppose she doesn't get a full dose due to poor technique? I know my hands trembled. Some fluid leaked out; the qualified nurse supervising had said it was nothing more than she would expect. Expect from an unqualified person who had never given an injection in their life before, or expect because that is what happens, some always leaks out? How often does a properly qualified person give Vera her injection?

I sign everything off and the supervisor ticks a couple of my boxes, first hurdle at least underway. How did Vera come to be in this state? Her notes only go back a few years. I need to know how she came into the system. The Ward Sister doesn't see why I can't get hold of her old notes if I want them.

A few days later her huge number of files are delivered on a wheeled trolley. I won't live long enough to read all this! She was first seen as quite a young child where she was described as *imbecilic*.

Idiot, imbecile, feeble-minded, moral imbecile and moron were formal classifications of intellectual capacity. In 1913 the definitions were tightened in law and covered by the Mental Deficiency Act:

The following classes of persons who are mentally defective shall be deemed to be defectives within the meaning of this Act: -

(a) Idiots; that is to say, persons so deeply defective in mind from birth or from an early age as to be unable to guard themselves against common physical dangers.

(b) Imbeciles; that is to say, persons in whose case there exists from birth or from an early age mental defectiveness not amounting to idiocy, yet so pronounced that they are incapable of managing themselves or their affairs, or, in the case of children, of being taught to do so.

(c) Feeble-minded persons; that is to say, persons in whose case there exists from birth or from an early age mental defectiveness not amounting to imbecility, yet so pronounced that they require care, supervision, and control for their own protection or for the protection of others, or, in the case of children, that they by reason of such defectiveness appear to be permanently incapable of receiving proper benefit from the instruction in ordinary schools;

(d) Moral imbeciles; that is to say, persons who from an early age display some permanent mental defect coupled with strong vicious or criminal propensities on which punishment has had little or no deterrent effect.

The categories were loosely associated with expected development in years, so an imbecile was someone with a mental age of three to seven years, but Vera would barely have been seven when she was diagnosed. She was described as unsuitable for schooling and now in her fifties (precise age uncertain) she has done nothing in terms of either life experience or education. Her claim to fame, it seems to me, is pincushion for random students.

Her notes do not make the timing clear, but if this was the early 1930s she would have been placed in Darenth Park. The Darenth School for Imbecile Children opened in 1878 to take in children from the overflowing London Orphanage in Clapton. More than five hundred children were moved in covered wagons. It wasn't easy to get a place in the Clapton orphanage; there were always far more children than places. There was lobbying on behalf of a child for the twice-yearly intake. To move five hundred orphans who were supposed to have learning difficulties sounds all very progressive, but it can't be true because it would be more children than the Clapton orphanage could hold in total. It also seems unlikely they all had learning difficulties.

As the children aged it seems their abilities deteriorated despite the training systems. Adults were also moved to the site, and it became known as The Darenth Asylum. A farm was set up (the Darenth Industrial Trading Colony). The men and boys worked on the farm while the girls were trained in cleaning and laundry duties. The place was practically self-sufficient, and in its heyday there were some 2,260 patients. Many wards had more than fifty inmates.

But they stopped admitting children in 1935, so it could be that Vera lucked out (or struck lucky depending on your point of view). My estimation would be that she should have been diagnosed by 1935 unless she is younger than she looks. Because I'm still only twenty-one everyone seems old to me. In 1959 they started taking children again, long past the time Vera could have benefitted from the training provided. These days Darenth is seriously decrepit and no one in their right mind would send a child there. Yet there are still some fifteen hundred lost souls at Darenth Park Hospital, around five hundred of which are children. I watch them play when I'm not in class. A lot of them are unusually pale and blond, like angels. Although it was agreed that Darenth should close in 1973, there is no sign of it happening.

The vastness of the place is difficult to describe. It stands like some dark, satanic mill from the hymn "Jerusalem" and is the prominent vista as you travel south through the Dartford Tunnel from Essex. Row after row of massive three and four-storey white-stone buildings, set in two compounds slightly offset from one another. Being white (dirty actually) doesn't make them any less imposing. The grounds make up an entire farm.

I don't know whether Vera's mother kept her home by choice or because she had no choice. On her mother's death, Vera was placed in various halfway houses, rotating between failed placements and mental institutions. The leap to a diagnosis of dementia praecox, which eventually became known as schizophrenia, doesn't seem to be at all clear. Again and again, I read words like "inadequate" in descriptions of this friendly, placid woman. She seems to have been sedated in some way for most of her life, but I don't see any reason why this might be.

Looking at her now it seems she could do with livening up rather than calming down. The fact she remembered me doesn't fit with the imbecile label. It could be argued the antipsychotic injections are doing their job – I wouldn't know. I can't find anyone on the staff who can remember anything other than a pleasant, plump woman without a life. Had she made it as a moron she may have had some kind of education. This term was reserved for those with the intellectual capacity of an eight-to-twelve-year-old. Moral imbeciles or morons were considered the most dangerous of the feebleminded as they could be likely to reproduce since they had poor morals!

Since I have such an interest in Vera I have been asked to take her to St Thomas Hospital in Lambeth for a dental appointment. This is a big deal. I am only a junior trainee and responsible for the care of Vera on a train journey that will take more than an hour and what will be – for her at least – a lengthy walk at the other end.

Or we could go by ambulance. Although I would like Vera to have the chance for a day out, the travelling time will be more than halved if we go by ambulance. In the end the responsibility seems too great, and I accept the offer of the ambulance. Shame on me; if I were older maybe, more secure in my ability, we could have had a day out in the city, lunch in a café perhaps.

Travelling through South London by ambulance sans lights and sirens is weird. You can't take in the views, there isn't any sense of direction or progress, and Vera is on a bed even though she isn't sick, just pleasant and placid and in need of a dental appointment.

The clinic is modern, lots of glass and steel. Vera plonks herself on a chair and leaves me to sort out the paperwork. I notice that there is a red tab on the top of the card that prefaces her notes. Across the top of the card in large capital letters it says SCHIZOPHRENIC. I'm not sure that has anything to do with her teeth.

We are reading magazines – at least I am; Vera looks at the pictures. We chat occasionally but we have been there much longer than I feel we should. I am the one getting agitated!

Eventually I crack and go to the reception desk. I explain that we have come a long way, we have an ambulance waiting and our appointment was an hour ago. I am told the appointment time is arbitrary; it's on a first come first served basis. That doesn't wash either, but I sit back down, carefully watching the box of files. I see the red tab getting closer to the front and then sure enough! Exactly as I suspected, the next nurse takes Vera's card and notes and shifts it to the back of the box. I leap from my seat like a pouncing tiger.

I think I state Vera's case loudly enough for the poor nurse to wish the ground would swallow her up. She stutters and stammers and apologises, and funnily enough it transpires we are next. Vera would have sat there all day, waiting patiently for her turn which would never have come. My blood is boiling.

The dentist works some magic. I don't watch – I'm not afraid of dentists, but the yuk factor is more than I can stand bearing in mind the ambulance had already made me feel queasy. Just as well we have our private transport though – Vera sleeps most of the way back. Mission accomplished.

Realistically the only time I get to read the old notes is after my shift has finished. Everyone is getting fed up with the trolley being in the way and I only have a couple of weeks left before I move to a new area. The old writing is so faded in some notes, it may as well have been written in invisible ink, and the scrawl that some people call handwriting is shocking. Some of the files have had more sun than others and the edges of the thin card holding the sheaths of paper crumble in my hands. The paper itself varies in quality over the years. Some has turned to dust. There is also water damage and even bits that have been eaten. I have read as far as the diagnosis switching from dementia praecox to schizophrenia – subtype: Catatonic.

This is something I know about from my studies. Emil Kraepelin came up with the term dementia praecox and he realised that there were many varieties of the disorder. He described a general decay and loss of mental efficiency, and a loss of mastery over volitional action. He had a sense that there could be much more to be discovered – he supposed around nine varieties. Given the childhood diagnosis of imbecility I couldn't see how Vera could have a general decay of mental efficiency since mental efficiency wasn't her star turn in the first place.

By the time I came to the nursing school we were down to four subtypes: hebephrenic, catatonic, paranoid and simple. Schizophrenia is complex, delusions, hallucinations, disorganised speech and / or behaviour and a lack of enthusiasm. Not everyone has every symptom, and Vera has nothing bar a lack of enthusiasm!

There are two variants of lists that are used to sort patients into labels by their symptoms: Diagnostic and Statistical Manual of Mental Disorders (DSM) and the International

Classification of Diseases (ICD). Basically they're books of medical cheat sheets – if the patient displays this symptom, then they have that disease. DSMIII has recently been published and so should be great, but I don't think the writers have ever seen a real patient because things are more complicated in the real world than they are on paper. ICD is put out by the World Health Organisation and covers physical disorders and some mental ones, while the DSM is specific to mental disorders and is produced by American psychiatrists. The latest DSM is supposed to provide consistency between the two manuals. Both are viewed with suspicion by coalface workers.

Catatonic schizophrenia has quite definitive symptoms according to my learning and is divided into positive symptoms of excited catatonia. Vera could not possibly fit into an excited category of anything. The negative type involves symptoms such as staring, mutism, waxy flexibility, echolalia or echopraxia. To my mind staring and mutism are symptoms of being bored skull-less – nothing to see and nothing to say. Waxy flexibility means you can put someone into a posture and they will stay there. For instance, if you raise their arm it stays in place instead of flopping down by their side. I wouldn't blame them if they punched you; I'm not going to try it. Echolalia and echopraxia are interesting; echolalia involves repeating a word or phrase you have just heard, literally being an echo. Echopraxia is the repetition of another's actions. If Vera did either of these things in the past – and I still haven't found any documented evidence – then the injections put paid to it. If your only activity is in the service of the nurse-training department as resident pincushion I can see why imitating others might be attractive. Co-opt someone else's life and call it your own.

All I see is a silent tragedy.

This makes everything sound very sad but the genuine care for her from the staff is the only solace I can take from this experience. The reputation of asylums in general has been sullied by various investigations inferring conditions and treatment are more like prisons. The grounds here are magnificent; Vera can take walks, visit the chapel and she is very welcome in the workshops though she struggles to do much.

I love the glass conservatory where the weaving takes place. There are some skilled souls here who make huge peacock rattan chairs. Rattan is made from a type of climbing palm tree imported from Asia. The work is intricate, and the chairs sell for big money. Patients living at Stone House full time are realistically the only ones likely to reach the skill level for these chairs. I have been tasked with making two child-sized chairs using a cheaper plastic substitute which is easier to use for the talentless. Even this is beyond my skill level but the first hasn't turned out too badly. I kept it to one colour, a sort of pale wheat shade, so any mistakes are less likely to show. My next one is going to be a combination of brown and the wheat colour. The weave will be the same chequered pattern, but any mistakes will really stand out. Weaving in the warm bright conservatory is so relaxing I could do it every day. I can see the attraction of living here!

Something else has happened that initially hadn't worried me. President Tito of Yugoslavia died last year. That was bad enough but things have become much worse – the country has been borrowing from both America and Russia on different terms and now can't afford to repay the debts to either. We have a holiday in Yugoslavia booked for September – the first time we have been abroad together – but the word on the street is there are armed guards all over the country and the dinar is worth nothing. The currency I did manage to get will barely buy us breakfast! We didn't need passports when we booked and now we do. We have been issued with temporary UK passports. The travel agent assures me the trip is safe – it is being able to afford to eat that is worrying me. I failed my driving test again and we can't afford more lessons, so we have to get someone to drive us to the airport.

Chapter 10: Mothers and Babes

The holiday in Yugoslavia wasn't a complete disaster. The weather was fabulous, but our money was worth nothing. You could put a pile of Yugoslav dinar on the bar and wrangle a drink from the barman because you were English, something the Germans couldn't do! The waiter at the hotel stole food from German breakfast plates and passed it to us for our lunch, knowing we couldn't afford any. We were alarmed by the guards with guns at the airport as they checked our temporary passports, but after that we never saw a soldier, nor a policeman, and people were literally walking around with wheelbarrows of cash.

Why I thought a lime green bikini would be a fashion statement over my milk-white skin and flat chest I have no idea. I could be seen for miles, especially since we had ended up next to a naturist beach where nothing but white ankle socks were all the rage. I'm not built for that!

—\/\/\—

Still, I am cheered up, well rested, and excited about this placement. But when I enter the Joyce Green MHU there is the most appalling smell that permeates the whole building. Surely it should be emptied and fumigated? Something has gone terribly wrong.

The unit has a male ward, and a female ward joined by a common dining and recreation room. The smell reaches every corner of it. The source is a bloke on a mattress on the floor of the male dormitory, amongst cigarette butts and cockroaches. He is dying. He poured petrol over himself and set fire to it on the beach in front of his girlfriend. She is in the female wing.

He was taken by ambulance to the Burn Unit directly from the beach, but he fought everyone who tried to help, and in the end the burns people refused to take him. Although the point of the 1959 Act (under which we are still labouring while the new code is sorted out) was to reduce compulsory treatment, there is still provision for this kind of emergency. Clearly he

79

must have *some* kind of treatment, so he is detained under the 1959 Act for fourteen days. He won't last fourteen days. He has been brought to the unit to die because his burns will become infected (have already judging by the smell), and he will die. No one can tend his wounds – we just hold him down to inject sedatives and painkillers. This is the worst thing I have ever experienced. His girlfriend watches over him and everyone in the unit will be forever haunted by the smell of burnt human flesh.

He is dead within the week. I have no idea why his girlfriend is still here – surely she would have wanted to go elsewhere unless she had some hope he would recover? She is mute, still in shock. If she didn't want to be within his dying stench she couldn't have told anyone.

It may be the way of the future but there is a stigma involved in being a patient here. It was never mentioned to me in the medical unit but plenty of the patients here tell me this is a plague hospital. They are referring to its use during outbreaks of smallpox, which just last year has been declared eradicated from the world. It is a long while since vaccination was stopped. I was vaccinated aged four because it was required for travel by boat to Australia when I was the daughter of ten-pound Poms in 1963.

Planning for Joyce Green as a smallpox hospital was already underway in 1893 but was delayed by arguments over its size, so when there was a severe outbreak in 1901 Joyce Green wasn't ready. Instead, that outbreak was catered for by the tents in the Darenth Marsh area, plus temporary buildings (Long Reach and The Orchard) that opened early in 1902. Between them these buildings could take 664 patients on top of the 300 in the tents.

Joyce Green eventually opened in 1903 to replace the smallpox ships, the *Atlas, Endymion* and *Castalia*, but in the end the hospital never saw any smallpox cases. They took patients with other infectious diseases, like scarlet fever, measles, diphtheria and whooping cough. The closest they came to smallpox was in 1918, when they housed over a thousand Russian troops that had come into contact with it. The Orchard was destroyed by fire in World War Two, and Long Reach was maintained with a skeleton staff until it closed in 1973. The buildings were destroyed in 1975 as part of the Thames flood barrier. It is astonishing – people's memories must be heritable because most of these current patients weren't even born when plagues were a problem. The recollection was most likely kept alive because fever nurses were still being trained here until the early 70s. Patients are doubly resistant to the notion of a mental health unit in the grounds of a hospital associated with contagious disease.

—∿—

I still haven't passed my driving test. Without lessons, I'm going to have to take the next test in the Triumph that we swapped the Honda for. The problem is that it will only go into first gear if it is at an absolute standstill. Stan reckons he will take it apart and see what the problem is. There's also a waitlist for the tests, but I've been told you can get a higher place if you're a nurse. So I will try that. And I have been advised to wear my uniform.

I know the rules of the road and have been riding bikes for years – I got my bike licence on the day of my seventeenth birthday. Perhaps that's the problem – I've fallen into bad habits. I failed the last test for turning into a gap in the traffic that was too small. Clearly it wasn't because I didn't smash into anything, but the tester said I forced the car I pulled in front of to slow down. I felt we had waited an embarrassing length of time already and were holding up the cars behind. Plus, the turn was at the top of a hill, so I was balanced on the clutch as it was.

—∿—

The MHU was opened in 1969 at the end of the western arm of the long outdoor corridors that are now covered overhead in glass but bare at the sides. There are two such corridors in the shape of a V. I can only describe the wards as pavilions coming off the corridors like veins on a leaf where the corridors are the midrib of each leaf. The wind blows across the corridors. I guess that it makes sense to have the MHU at an end – at least the patients don't commonly arrive on a gurney.

Figure 4. Joyce Green (Fever) Hospital, near Dartford

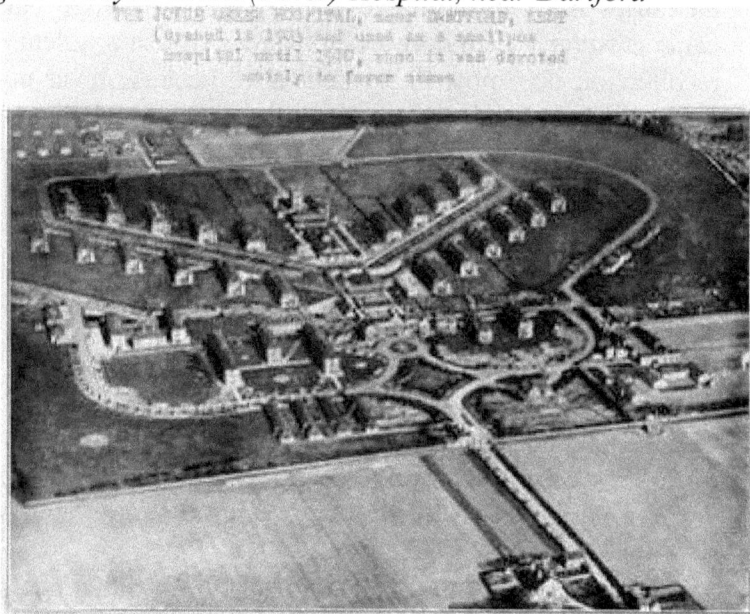

Credit: Wellcome Library, London. Powell, Allan Published: 1930. The MHU was opened in 1969 and not shown in this photograph.

Once the bins are emptied, causing a massive reduction in acute beds, this unit will host all the acutely mentally unwell in the area. What especially attracts me is the mother and baby unit. This area of psychiatry fascinates me. I don't have a baby so I don't know what it feels like, but I do know pregnancy and birth can have serious effects on some mothers. I'm aware the couple we bought our house from had problems.

I watch Sister in the darkened room set aside for mothers (with or without babies). Currently there is only one patient. Sister sits sewing rhythmically and rocking in a chair as the patient falls asleep for the first time in days. Other staff care for the baby. This mother has become so exhausted. She was found shopping, noticed because the groceries were piled on top of the baby in the pram as if he wasn't in it. Her husband had feared things weren't going well but didn't know what to do or where to get help. He had to go to work to pay the bills, and her mother lives too far away. How would the average man even know there *was* help? Mine wouldn't have a clue!

Before the week is out another young mother has arrived with her baby. The baby is six weeks old and the young mum seems happy. She doesn't report feeling at all depressed, she says she doesn't hear voices or have any unusual thoughts but doesn't know what she is supposed to do. If I were a mother at sixteen I wouldn't know what to do either. The family insist she can't cope, which is a bit different from not knowing what to do. This isn't her family. I don't know how her family fit in, but this young couple are living with *his* parents. He is seventeen and his mother seems supportive, but exhausted. I suspect she is doing too much, and the sixteen-year-old mother doesn't see the need to pull her weight. A simple issue, so we send the family home for a rest and keep the mother and baby. We quickly find another problem – she can't make up the infant formula to the concentration the baby needs. He is quite a placid little chap, an ideal baby.

We draw pictures of scoops and cups of water for her, but counting isn't in her skill set either. She has been here for six weeks, and we can't find anything wrong with her, the baby, the family, or the living conditions. There are mothers who can neither read nor count and they manage. All the other patients, male and female, have been helping in one way or another – everyone has an opinion! Eventually Sister organises a psychologist.

We don't usually see psychologists in the hospital – in fact I have never seen one, though they have been guest speakers at the nursing school. I have had thoughts about training – or at least looking into training – to be a psychologist, now I've found that I am not the waste of space my school report would indicate. Everything happens behind closed doors though; an interested student nurse is not welcome. So I have no idea what went on in there – but the report was swift and significant. This young woman is never going to be capable of caring for her baby.

Her IQ (Intelligence Quotient) is sixty. I know a little bit about IQ. The eleven-plus – an unpopular test for eleven-year-olds – is a variation on the IQ and divides children into academic, technical or vocational categories. Thereafter the students are schooled accordingly. It was sort of phased out in 1976, long after I sat it, though it still persists in my neck of the woods. My understanding – and I'm not sure where this came from – is that the school entrance exam for the posh(ish) school I was eventually thrown out of required a minimum IQ score of one hundred and thirty points to get to the interview and entry-exam stage. One hundred and thirty can't be that smart because otherwise I wouldn't have got kicked out at fifteen. Either that or I was smart at ten and got dimmer which, considering I have tried frying my brains, is also possible. Sister tells me one hundred and thirty *is* smart and I must have got dimmer – or there was a mistake calculating the results!

The psychologist's report poses a significant problem for this family. A score of sixty indicates mild mental retardation, which might not sound so bad, but caring for a baby is quite complex. This is not a problem dealt with by a mental health unit. Sitting in on the family meeting, I watch it slowly dawn on the grandparents that they have, in addition to a son who can't keep his trousers zipped, acquired a daughter who will not function as an independent adult without a great deal of training and support. Plus a grandchild who may be good-natured because he doesn't have much going on upstairs either! He is quite likely the result of a quick fumble, which is no basis for a lasting relationship. As the meeting draws to a close, the mother of the boy with the trouser problem looks as if she has been hit on the head with a cricket bat. I am not surprised.

–∿–

84

An elderly lady is admitted from the orthopaedic ward. The orthopaedic doctor has truly wound Sister up by diagnosing schizophrenia.

"What does a bone doctor know?" she yells, "I won't tell him how to fix broken bodies if he leaves broken minds to the professionals." It is worse than that; he has used the 1959 Mental Health Act to do it! Her bones have mended, and she wants to go home. He must have managed to get another doctor to agree to this because two are required under the terms of the Act. This lady is elderly but physically fit, her memory is sharp, and she can count back from a hundred in sevens; you try it! The only thing at issue is the way the fall came about. Past tense, fall that has already happened. What is it about a belief over a past incident that could constitute an emergency under the terms of the Act? The paperwork says she has a *fixed delusion*. She believes she was spreadeagled down the stairs in her block of flats by skiers. Her notes plainly state that she fell down the stairs.

"Does it matter?" I ask myself aloud. Sister says it is misuse of the Act and the poor old duck has not had a say in the matter because it is standard practice not to tell anyone that they have any rights. It all makes Sister really riled up! Technically the old lady should be here for fourteen days to treat her for a belief that does not affect her day-to-day functioning but sounds weird. If "weird" was something you could be locked up for, then most of my friends would be put away. Definitely most of my family!

Some students turn up to see the old lady at visiting time. They want to talk to Sister privately before the visit. They are clearly nervous. As they should be! They sheepishly admit that they bought skis for a winter holiday. After a few beers it seemed like a great idea to try the skis out on the communal stairs... They had visited her in the broken bone ward, taken flowers and grapes but hadn't admitted the full extent of their involvement. Now, with the stakes raised, they had to confess.

Figure 5. Treponema pallidum

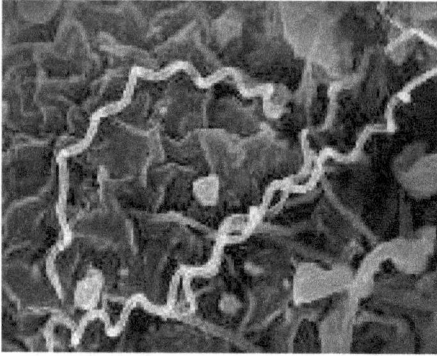

Electron micrograph of Treponema pallidum, the bacteria that cause syphilis. Several spiral-shaped bacteria have been highlighted. Credit: NIAID 2023

Chapter 11: A Wanton Lifestyle

A bloke has collapsed in the corridor outside Long Stay –
Male. I have no idea where he is from – this is an evening shift
so he could be a visitor. We drag him onto a bed and four of us
perform CPR for more than an hour. We are not allowed to
stop without the say so of a doctor. Since there isn't a doctor
in this hospital, one must be dragged in from elsewhere. A taxi
is needed because this *elsewhere* doctor doesn't drive, and by
the time he arrives, the four of us are almost as dead as the
patient.

If he had gone for a walk and collapsed on the other side of
the lake, then he would have been found dead in the morning.
As it is he was brutalised by four reasonably strong women for
more than an hour and two wards were deprived of care. On
the plus side he will have had more kisses than he probably
had in his entire life. It demonstrates very clearly how
ludicrous these uniforms are though. We had to practically
bare our backsides, hitching them up to kneel on the bed due
to the narrowness of the skirts. He would have stood a better
chance had we left him on the floor anyway.

The guys on Long Stay really need minimal care. There are
mostly shared rooms, some four to a room, so more privacy
than Male Admission. The patients are usually out during the
day; the evening is about dinner, medication and bed. All of
that has been disrupted by the dead guy in the corridor whose
name I do not even know. The brothers who got the police taxi
early on in my training have graduated to Long Stay Male.
Mostly the admission units discharge people home. It is rare
these days to shift to a long stay ward, especially considering
almost everyone is a voluntary patient.

We are supposed to know where everyone is, but it really
isn't possible. This makes handover to the next shift a bit of a
mire. It occurs to me – if we accept responsibility for someone
who hasn't been seen since breakfast and then they turn up
dead, who is responsible? Perhaps responsible isn't the right
word; if someone were killed then the staff here are not

responsible in the murderous sense, but wouldn't they be accountable in some way?

I need to understand these things because my ward management assessment will be here. It wouldn't be my first choice, but it has to be somewhere, and I want to undertake the patient care practical on female geriatrics so I can bath someone. It's the simplest kind of care I can do without risking too much of a cock-up. Technically I have eighteen months to complete four practical assessments. It sounds long enough but I'm beginning to feel pressured. Traditionally the teaching assessment is last, which I want to save for Female Admission because a friend of mine will be working there then. Mabledon is too hectic for ward management, and I can't do patient care on a ward where the patients (residents – I don't feel they are patients) barely receive any care at all!

—∿—

Wilf should be in Male Geriatrics. He is still here in Long Stay because it is his home. He is also so sweet the staff don't want him to move on. He catches flies and eats them. He also swallows coins and has a few lodged in his lungs. Not ideal. His mum comes every Sunday. She is in her nineties; she brings a silver tea set and little cakes which she sets up on a three-tier cake stand. Everything is carefully placed on a white tablecloth. She doesn't let him eat flies while they have afternoon tea. Usually he can barely sit still, but he does for her. Wilf has GPI (General Paralysis of the Insane) the result of untreated syphilis. He is a bit of an enigma because he should be dead. Before the advent of penicillin syphilis was fatal.

Wilf has neurosyphilis, where the bacterium *Treponema pallidum* has got into his central nervous system. Initially symptoms of GPI were thought to be due to alcohol and a wanton lifestyle. It was associated with soldiers and railway workers but not vicars. Men may not have any symptoms of syphilis. Even if Wilf had known he'd contracted what was called the lady's disease, early treatments were either mercury inhalation (horribly toxic), or inducing a fever with malaria.

The malaria could then be controlled by quinine. He was likely to die anyway. Yes, this is true: people were given malaria to raise their body temperature (pyrotherapy) to cure syphilis. Julius Wagner-Jauregg won a Nobel prize for discovering this treatment! Psychiatrists don't often win Nobel prizes. He wasn't such a great guy because he killed quite a number of WWI soldiers that he thought were malingering by giving them extreme ECT.

That wasn't his only claim to fame. He also sterilised people who had schizophrenia because he believed it was caused by excessive masturbation. Presumably this was in males only because in women hysteria was cured by inducing an orgasm, which plenty of doctors practised! Although pyrotherapy was claimed to cure syphilis, most of the patients relapsed within a few years and died. Now GPI is rare because anyone with it should have died long ago. Wilf never got that message and, complete with the coins in his lungs, the fly diet and intractable psychosis, he looks like he will go on forever.

I can't move on from syphilis without mentioning the Tuskegee study. It was supposed to last six months but was extended to forty years between 1932 and 1972 in Alabama, USA. Six hundred sharecroppers were enticed by the offer of free medical care into what was supposed to be a six-month study. Three hundred and ninety-nine of them had latent syphilis but were never told. Of the two hundred and one control members of the study that did **not** have syphilis at the start, some found out they were positive later when they tried to enlist in the army. They were prevented from accessing treatment by the Tuskegee study board, even though, as a control group, they were no longer useful. The participants were subject to diagnostic procedures and ineffective treatment despite penicillin being widely available as a standard treatment from at least 1947. Twenty-eight of them died from syphilis, one hundred died from complications related to syphilis, forty of the patients' wives were infected, and nineteen children were born with congenital syphilis. The funding had been withdrawn many years before the study was officially ended, but the point is that treatment was never going to be offered anyway, the men were duped. A medical panel found in 1972 that the study was medically unjustified and in 1974 a class action awarded US$10 million in compensation and treatment to the surviving participants and their families.

Some of the Long Stay residents are the craftsmen working in the glass conservatory on the peacock chairs, some go off to work, and some who are retired visit friends or family. One bloke goes off on a bicycle every morning to work and is supposed to return after lunch. It is ironic that he rides everywhere because he was admitted in the 1940s for stealing a bicycle. He has been here ever since, but today he hasn't come back, and I don't know what to put on the handover sheet. As a student I'm not responsible, but Charge is missing. I do need to find him; he isn't on the ward, but this place is a rabbit warren. There are grand staircases which we all use, but back stairs as well, presumably for servants when people paid to stay here. I don't want to leave the ward, yet I feel I should find him. Both of the long stay wards are on the first floor, and there is a large space between them, but I have never explored it. I think it is a lounge for the doctors. There are more back stairs going up yet again, presumably to attic rooms – perhaps staff accommodation? I have no idea if there is anything up there now.

I push through the heavy glass doors and they close quickly behind me, propelling me into the room. The lounge is empty. I mean *really* empty – there is carpet, but nothing else. My shoelace is undone. I can't ignore it; being a klutz, I *will* trip, so I bend down to fix it.

Someone enters. I sense they are bigger than average, and looking up, I see tan corduroy legs. Raising my eyes further, I note the waistband is too high, topped by two checked shirts in different checks and unbuttoned more than is usual, plus an old person's cardigan. He doesn't seem old, but the dress code shouts crazy. He has sandals without socks. No one in England wears sandals without socks in winter. He isn't a doctor and suddenly I'm tense.

"You shouldn't be here," he said. "This is private territory." He has an accent. American? Canadian? Canadians can be a bit touchy if anyone suggests they are from America. Either would be unusual around here.

I'm fumbling with an octopus of loops that's laughing at me and now the outer fabric of the lace has parted from the core – muddling things further. I should stand up, but if I need to run then I want the laces fixed. Kneeling on the floor in front of a giant is a vulnerable position and my heart is pounding in my ears.

"You gotta a Walkman?" the voice booms. It almost seems like a demand rather than a query. I bought one for Stan, a Christmas present. The sound is brilliant, but he carries batteries wrapped together with tape, like sticks of dynamite peeking out of his pocket. The battery life of the device itself is hopeless.

Answering honestly, "I don't have one," I scramble to my feet, laces in some kind of knot.

A voice from behind confirms that I should not be here. Spinning around, I see there is another extra-large human being. I don't know who these people are – the door was neither locked nor labelled.

"Let her be on her way, Chay, you have no need of her."

I stand stock still; time is doing the same.

Eventually the guy with the accent says, "Be on your way, I have no use for you."

I don't need telling twice.

Who are these people? I have stopped caring where Charge is. I run back to the ward and write on the sheet that Bicycle Guy is unaccounted for.

The afternoon shift insist I stay. They are not prepared to take over with someone unaccounted for. Still no sign of Charge. Our errant resident eventually turns up without remorse or even a vague excuse about where he has been, and I leave. The next day Charge claims to have gone off sick. If I am in training for my ward management assessment, then it would be courteous if the staff let me know where they are!

Rampton

The nursing school has booked all the students across the years for a coach trip. We are supposed to be supernumerary, but the wards are outraged about the sudden loss of slave labour.

Our coach trip is to Rampton, a secure hospital opened in 1912 to take overspill from Broadmoor, the country's main secure hospital. Originally an asylum for the criminally mentally ill, it closed temporarily at the end of 1919 and reopened as an institution for mental defectives rather than lunatics. Some of the women considered to have more hope were kept on and trained for domestic service. Eventually the hospital was open for men and women with either mental illness or intellectual disability who were in need of secure care.

At around 160 miles, it should be a three-hour journey. Except the M1 is closed somewhere north. So far, we have been more than four hours on a coach without a toilet. It would be fair to say that tempers are frayed! We would rather have gone to Broadmoor anyway, which is a high security psychiatric hospital *and* a hundred miles closer!

Things get worse if that is possible. Because we're two hours late, our hosts decide we should miss most of the tour and concentrate on the treatment of the intellectually disabled. This is not something covered in our training (although I do not know everyone on the coach, so it is quite possible there *are* students for the qualification here). It is quite disturbing to most of us because these people are seriously without hope. Our aspirations rely on hope – our patients are destined to get better and lead normal lives. Even the institutionalised are supposed to be leaving care and living in the community. Well, that's the grand plan though I still see no evidence of that other than the already mentioned booting out of my dear Nan's friends for the crime of pregnancy, which is not an ongoing condition.

Rampton has recently been through the mill with a documentary last May called *Rampton, The Secret Hospital* that suggested ill treatment. A highly disputed investigation reported the patients here have less dignity than a family pet. The tables are bolted to the floors because one of the nurses was hit with a trestle table and sustained a broken back. The people on *display* today have no idea which way is up.

I'm disturbed by the sight of a woman with clubbed hands and feet and without a neck. I watch as she is shifted from her empty room to a wire-fenced garden across the corridor, which is cut off by wooden partitions installed for the very reason of getting her out of the room. A fire hydrant is turned on her to *swoosh* her into the garden without risk of her being within reach of another human... ever. Her food gets shoved through a hole in the bottom of the door. We are told she has five X chromosomes (women usually have two; five is very rare). They say it is the result of her mother having an X-ray during pregnancy. I find this unlikely but then I don't know everything. I do know this isn't a life.

We go home dissatisfied. Some of the boys are slightly interested; they have been told if you qualify as a registered psychiatric nurse then you can get a charge nurse job in a hospital for the intellectually handicapped. This seems appalling to me – it is quite a different speciality – but they are looking at the pay difference between Staff nurse and Charge.

So, we had a dreadful journey with a grumpy driver. We didn't see or talk to anyone useful, and my bladder hasn't coped. Yet the next morning we find things have become worse than we could ever have imagined. The coach driver went home, put his family under the table, and shot them.

—∿—

For my next trick I'm cycling to Norfolk. I finally have a car licence, but I don't want to drive, I feel the need for a challenge, an adventure of sorts. It is my brother's 21st birthday and my pushbike has never seen any action; to be truthful, I'm down in the dumps. I bought a track suit to give the appearance of a seasoned cyclist. It is more than 150 miles.

The first night will be at Stan's mum's place. Then on to Cambridge where I'll stay at the university. Finally, to my Mum and Dad's pig farm. The weather is predicted to be dreadful, but I don't care. I need a break. I have also signed up to an Open University course, Social Science (D102), it is a full year extramural course, you have to watch TV in the early hours of the morning after regular night time TV has shut down and attend a summer school in September, my mind needs to be completely occupied all of the time.

Chapter 12: Spending Spree

When I cycled to Norfolk in foul weather and the worst tracksuit, I discovered how kind people could be. Loads of people offered to help or give me a lift even though I had a bike. I declined them all. Yes, I was freezing and wet the whole time. Yes, my tracksuit was so heavy it built muscles on the spindles I call legs. But it got me out of my funk.

We had deep snow on the day of Roy's birthday. Stan came up on his motorbike. I couldn't have gone back with him because of the bicycle so I caught the train home. Very brave of me. Although we have the car we bought after the Honda threw me off when the back wheel locked up, Stan still doesn't have a licence so he can't drive it without me.

That weekend we decided the car we'd thought was a good swap for a dodgy bike was actually a lemon the dealer was glad to unload. We also agree I should have a brand-new motorbike. I choose Italian – known for their quality. A Moto Guzzi V50. This is a 500cc with twin cylinders in a 'V' formation. I don't have to reach the brake lever because the front and back brakes are linked. This has been a problem for ages. The front brake on the Honda had long since seized where it had never been used because my stubby fingers couldn't reach the lever. The Guzzi also has a drive shaft, so no more mucky chains. It doesn't have a kick start either so my mass – which has grown to fifty kilos on account of the cake – can't break it. And it has a car battery, so no more running down the road with a flying leap to bump-start it. I think they only come in red.

—᭚—

Two of us are tasked with spending as much of the interest accrued in the accounts of the wealthy patients as we can, as fast as we can. It sounds like a scam, but it will be absorbed into the hospital coffers come the end of the tax year if we don't. The Asylums Act in 1845 made the taxpayer responsible for asylum construction – a social safety net. In 1890 an Act permitted the admission of private patients. Stone House had recently bought the small Stone Lodge Farm, so they could advertise fresh food, fresh air and outdoor activities. In 1892 they started taking private patients (separated from the paupers) at one pound per week. This led to expansion and improvements – even electricity!

By 1906 fully half the patients were fee paying and they were turning people away. Most of the ladies here on Female Geriatrics will have been here since those heydays when families could rid themselves of an embarrassing problem. Some are from well-known families. As it is, the hospital occasionally benefits from the death of patients whose relatives cannot be traced. Some are in possession of a fortune. A few of the relatives organise escorted holidays for their loved ones... not so loved that they get visited, but loved enough to make the money go somewhere before the tax man has it.

Not many of them do more than walk around the grounds and visit the chapel. There is a splendid dayroom with ornately decorated ceilings and cornices, but often they will sit in the corridor. It is easily the width of an average lounge, and because it is along the outside of the building it has the same massive windows as elsewhere. The corridor is flooded with sunshine even this early in the year. The patients entertain themselves making comments to anyone passing through. They have their favourites who will stop and banter – porters, nurses, cleaners, even the lesser spotted visitor! Male and female hospital wards are beyond the double doors. This is where these old ducks will end their days, in the decrepit later additions at the end of the hospital. Because they are of retirement age they aren't required to attend occupational therapy, so they entertain themselves. They would have made up the bulk of the audience at the hospital shop where Oonagh entertained them with her dancing. What has been seen cannot be unseen.

Our shopping doesn't involve the High Street and shopping trolleys; we are ordering from a catalogue. When I was a child, we called these our "wish and want" books, though very rarely were we allowed to order anything. So this is exciting – until it isn't. Colourful curtains and counterpanes, televisions in every room – we are struggling to think of anything novel. We did think about the modern continental quilts – I have one of my own, not being keen on bedmaking –, but we felt it was a step too far for the ladies here. Anyway, the tog-rating business bamboozled us! The only togs I know are the ones you swim in.

The last lot of curtains and counterpanes aren't really worn out but are a bit dingy, a sort of duck-egg-blue fake silk (the hospital wash wouldn't cope with real silk). We have gone for brightly coloured flowery bedspreads and tried to get curtains to match in crisp cotton and linen. The gaudy seventies-style stuff wouldn't work in the Victorian, faux Tudor setting. I'm not sure about the flowers but they are cheerful. Not all the patients are wealthy, but the love will be spread; everyone will get something. To be truthful I feel that the hospital benefits more from this than the patients. If the hospital absorbed all this interest into their own coffers and used it to fix stuff that needs fixing, such as the lifting gear in Female Hospital or replaced the cracked lino then the money wouldn't have to be spent in a rush. It is because the canny ward Sister knows that no one will ever see it if it gets left.

—∿—

Amelia was one of the women admitted to the bar after the Sex Disqualification (Removal) Act 1919 meant that gender could not be used as a barrier to several professions and to university entry. Some universities did allow women entry earlier (London) but would only give them a "Certificate of Proficiency", and some universities (notably Cambridge) refused to award women a degree until 1948 regardless of the law. Of course, women needed a degree to enter the bar which they had been prevented from attaining so it wasn't until 1921 that the first women could become lawyers. Amelia qualified in 1926 but didn't last long after poking her tongue out at a judge (I have no idea why), he sent her to the County Lunatic Asylum and she never left. She is an imposing woman, approaching six foot and quite muscular. She races around the place, mostly chasing little Lita, a non-verbal Jewish girl – the staff call her a girl; she is in her seventies but looks much younger and is tiny and child-like. She clearly annoys the hell out of Amelia.

Amelia is the woman that I need to get on the good side of because she is the one I will be bathing for my patient care assessment. Bathing is about the simplest sort of care I can demonstrate, but to make it a challenge I have chosen one of the more difficult women to deal with. She's scary but some of the ladies here are an absolute hoot! Old Ma Cummings is a comedian; I have no idea what she did to get here but she has everyone in stitches. She has a swollen belly and tells everyone that she is pregnant, but it is regularly drained. I would say that there is a reason for the fluid building up, but no one seems worried. My understanding is that once you are past sixty no one takes your health seriously. Keeping people comfortable but not doing too much investigation is what it looks like to me. One of the general nurses doing her psych stint in Female Admission told me that even if you rock up to Accident and Emergency in an ambulance, you won't get serious treatment if you are old.

What I do notice is that these women look mad even though they behave reasonably well (apart from Amelia). Old Ma Cummings tells me that it's because of the drugs. She is talking about the neuroleptics (such as Chlorpromazine, Haloperidol, Pimozide) which aren't new, but were supposed to be wonder drugs that would result in everyone leaving the hospital. She describes how she used to go shopping without anyone knowing she was mad. Now she doesn't go anywhere because people stare at her, and even though she is a clown rather than mad, she is angry –, or she would be if she weren't such an optimistic character. What she is referring to are the side effects of the miracle medications. They might stop hallucinations but have the side effect of tardive dyskinesia. This affects mostly facial muscles, resulting in continuous tongue movements, lip smacking and puckering, grimacing, blinking, and a type of walk / gait that simply makes you look mad.

I'm thinking about where these ladies might go when the bins are emptied. Lita could be alright in an old folk's home and Ma Cummings if she lives long enough. A few, principally Amelia, wouldn't be tolerated anywhere I can think of. If the most able – or realistically the least troublesome – residents move out first, then the hospital will be left with a higher concentration of seriously sick or badly behaved patients. The best and most qualified nurses will also be on that first outward wave because they will be in demand. I'm concerned that a glimpse into my future shows that inexperienced and lesser qualified staff like me, will be stuck in crumbling buildings with broken patient hoists, dodgy lino, and the very worst patients.

—∧∧—

Our original class was six, but the two Mauritian boys doing two years to move from enrolled to registered have recently finished and got lucrative jobs as Charge Nurses at Darenth Park. They have no knowledge of intellectual impairment. Darenth is desperate enough that it doesn't matter. Mike, the Liverpudlian with glasses even thicker than mine, intends going there and so does Geoff, who seems a bit immature for psychiatry; maybe he would be better at Darenth. I guess he has time to mature – boys are a bit slow.

Then there is Joan. She is doing the full three years even though she is already a qualified enrolled nurse. I don't know why the difference. She is well meaning but like a scared rabbit caught in the headlights. I wouldn't want to work with her – she fluffs around in a mild panic the whole time.

We also have various transients join our classes. One of those is Terry, a friend of Geoff's. I'm not sure how or why he has joined our merry band, but he is creepy. His arms are too short and his fingers are stubby, he is slightly plump and sweaty, he has curly hair, and the sweat makes the curls stick to the side of his head. I don't like to feel this way, – I guess he can't help it – but whenever I'm around him I feel mildly nauseous. He isn't finishing with us though.

I would like to go to Joyce Green and specialise with the post-natal patients; I really enjoyed it. My concern is that without at least a general nurse registration, ideally both Registered Mental Nurse (RMN) and Registered General Nurse (RGN), I wouldn't stand a chance.

Today we have an admission. This is unheard of, or almost unheard of. The lady seems to be resigned to being here and aware that people from this ward don't generally leave. They get shifted to Female Hospital or die. They don't move back to Long Stay which would be the usual source of the people who end up here. It used to be the overspill from Female Admission that saw patients move to Long Stay. To make room for them they would move the oldest – or most geriatric I should say, because date of manufacture doesn't determine age of decrepitude. These days patients from Female Admission are much more likely to go home rather than to Long Stay. Even Het (Henrietta) is staying in Long Stay to die where she knows everyone rather than be shifted. She is getting more and more unsteady from Huntington's chorea, and more paranoid. It is top of my list of the worst ways to die (aside from burning buildings and plane crashes).

The new patient has ten children, and I ask Sister why she needs a place like this. I don't think I am being unreasonable – surely five weeks each wouldn't be too much to ask?

Sister turns the question around. "Why do you think none of her children will care for her, for even five weeks a year?"

I ponder this question. She doesn't have a history of mental illness, so surely an old folk's home would be better than this? I don't know how she has a bed. Her GP has described her as depressed... but aren't we all?

It quickly transpires that she is a mean, nasty battle-axe without a redeeming feature. She has nothing good to say about anyone and manages to upset old Ma Cummings and get chased by Amelia. Amelia doesn't exactly talk (although she can), she just throws obscenities and general growls, but she is not about to let someone else throw their weight about. The thing is that Amelia is genuinely mad and may very well beat the new lady senseless. I don't want Amelia riled up because I have my plans passed and I'm about to demonstrate the care that I can provide by bathing one of the most difficult patients in the building.

Arriving early, I take Amelia a cup of tea in bed. A treat because the usual routine is out and shower for those who are able and no tea until breakfast. I want her in the best mood. I remind her about the relaxing bath and am surprised that she has remembered. Instead of a bout of swearing she points out that a relaxing bath should be at the end of the day. She has a point, but I can only be assessed on day shift. I brought some bubble bath that smells of strawberries. I get her to smell it.

"I'm not having that in the bath, I'll smell like a fucking tart, like Lita. I'll kill her if she comes in!"

I reassure her that she will have the bathroom to herself. The bathrooms have two baths, back-to-back, so tap end backing onto the tap end of the other bath (cheaper) and you would be facing away from the other person. I could possibly be in the same bath with a very good friend. A strange person, in more ways than one, in a double bath situation beggars belief. I have arranged that no one, other than the Sister grading my skills, will be in there. All I have to do is get her there. I leave her drinking tea.

Sister watches me run the bath, complete with bubbles because whatever Amelia says about the smell – they will keep her amused, and I test the temperature of the water. I go to fetch Amelia. It could all go wrong right here because if she refuses then she is much too big for me to fight with, but everything is going smoothly. She even gets her own nightdress off, curious about the bubbles – the strawberry smell is barely discernible. The bath is quite deep; usually there isn't much water to prevent drowning, but I won't be taking my eyes off her for a second and I want it to be a real treat. I have even put her day clothes and towels on the radiator to warm. There are two large radiators hung on the adjacent wall, one for each bath. The baths though, are too close to the wall and there isn't enough room between the bath and the radiator. Many of the ladies could do with assistance from each side to get out of the deep Victorian baths and I am probably the only staff member small enough to fit. Even then I could get a burnt bum from the radiator.

She sinks into the bath, allowing the water to wash over her, and plays with the bubbles. She lets me wash her and scrub her back. I am going to smash this assessment. Until it is time to get out. That's when she tells us both to "fuck off" and starts to splash us, using her large hands as a scoop.

We back off as she refuses to get out. The water is now tepid, and if she runs the hot tap the bath is in danger of overflowing. It does have a vent to take off excess water, but in my mind it will be blocked after a hundred years without being used. I will flood the place and be in deep trouble.

I must think like a registered nurse on a busy ward. Leaping forward and plunging my arm into the water at the tap end, I pull out the plug. She is slow to react, and her thump misses me. The water drains away, and Amelia is lying in an empty bath and still refusing to move – despite the attraction of warm knickers. I am tempted to leave her to it – after all, she is responsible for herself for most of the day – but there is always the chance she could slip and bang her head.

Sister suggests we move to the bathroom corner, leaving Amelia to either freeze or get out. The room is big enough for some privacy and whatever Sister has to say, I can take it.

She tells me right out I have passed the assessment, so I relax. However, she has a point to make. The enrolled nurses, who have been here a hundred years (her words not mine), would have put Amelia in a tepid shallow bath – my mistake was making it too nice. She agrees that warm knickers are a reasonable luxury. She gave me ten out of ten for being quick-witted enough to pull the plug out and extra points for electing to bath Amelia in the first place. Meanwhile, Amelia has got herself out of the bath, made a rudimentary job with the towel, and dressed herself, intent on breakfast and Lita baiting.

Chapter 13: Idly Curious

I'm running past the "Keep off the Grass" sign as fast as I can when I hear a shout:

"WALK – we don't want things to go wrong!"

For a second I'm confused; they can't know the content of my message. Mary's grandchild isn't going to be any less dead, no matter my pace, so I slow to a trot. Then I realise they are concerned about my pregnancy – the notion enhanced by my beloved pinafore dress. This dress was my first purchase after I persuaded Mum I could choose my own clothes. She was convinced I would buy something outrageous, but this dress is the second most sensible fashion choice I have ever made. It is black needle-cord with a fitted quilted bodice. The cotton fabric of the bodice is black with tiny, brightly coloured flowers that are also repeated along the top of the patch pockets on the skirt.

It is great to run in. Not that I am a runner – far from it but it is a joy to be *able* to run. I have complained about the pain in my bones since I was about seven. Growing pains, apparently, what SHIT. I haven't grown as much as I would have liked, and the pain is crippling. It isn't constant, and I have tried to see if it links to food, to my period or to anything at all. I have kept a diary of its coming and going for years to no avail. Currently, it has mysteriously disappeared – the pain not the diary!

The pinafore dress *would* hide a bump but in this case there is nothing to see. Attempts at pregnancy have already been a disaster and while it isn't confirmed yet, this time I am truly hopeful; this is why my colleagues don't want me to run.

We have most of the Mabledon mob at Leeds Castle on an outing. We had started to spread out when a voice came over the sound system: "Will someone from Mabledon Hospital please call at the visitor's centre. There is an urgent message."

I am sent, being the least useful and most dispensable staff member. But the message isn't for me, the most junior and temporary of colleagues, but for Mary, one of the registered nurses, strong and bold. I can't be the one to deliver news like this. I run because I want rid of it as quickly as possible. It won't make any difference – dead is dead.

I blurt it out, in a poorly prepared huff and puff that makes me even less understandable. "Robert died during a seizure."

Consequently it takes a while for everyone to work out the magnitude of my statement.

We have come to the castle by coach, so Mary is stuck here while we round everyone up. This takes effort and quite some explaining. No one wants to go; it is a splendid sunny day and even if castles aren't your thing, Leeds Castle is beautiful. It covers two islands in a lake formed by the River Len. It was built by, and named after, a Saxon chief in 857 though this isn't the original wooden building. The castle has morphed over the years and was transformed in 1519 by Henry VIII for his then wife, Katherine of Aragon. The castle is so attractive it has popped up on film sets since the 1940s.

Most of the patients have a decent grasp of what has happened but they, like me, don't know what to do or say. I bury myself in the task of hunting down the stragglers.

Mary explains her daughter had taken Robert to hospital a couple of times recently because she thought there was something wrong. But he had no history of epilepsy. Certainly no one expected him to die.

The coach trip is grim. Made worse because from gut-wrenching pains and a dampness in my pants I know my period has started. Not wanting to ask the driver to stop, I curl up in my seat and try not to sob.

I still feel pregnant.

I don't know what to do. We have been making a concerted attempt for some time. We even tried using gravity to help (upside down on the stairs). We'd listened to a radio programme once about infertility. The expert claimed 1% of people he saw in his clinic were *doing it wrong*. That takes some thought.

In ancient Egypt a woman would pee on wheat and barley seeds over several days. If the barley grew, it indicated she was pregnant with a boy child. If the wheat grew, it was a girl. If neither grew, then there was no pregnancy. I don't think there is any evidence the sex of a child could be determined this way, but science does show the urine of a pregnant woman will promote seed growth. There are various claims throughout the ages about pee specialists who could detect pregnancy through colour, cloudiness, the presence of crystals or the numbers of bacteria. It wasn't until the 1920s that scientists recognised a specific hormone (human chorionic gonadotropin – hCG) was found only in pregnant women.

Because the idly curious didn't need to know if they were pregnant or not, and the service was already overstretched by testing for medical reasons, tests were initially not widely available. Demand for testing increased following the thalidomide disaster of the 1950s and rubella in the 1960s. During the early 1970s a home testing kit became available. Although it wasn't simple – there were warnings it was unreliable and not recommended for the average punter. As a sixteen-year-old I had gone to a proper clinic. They cocked it up by ignoring the words *soap-free container* in the instructions. This is what they told me when they contacted me to apologise. Too late, since I had dropped four tabs of acid and drunk four pints of Guinness by then. Celebrating the negative test. The sequelae of this I will probably take to my grave.

Now, in the 1980s, a pregnancy test kit is easily available but there is still a legacy regarding their reliability. So I'd decided to go to my GP. The problem with the GP is they often send a urine sample away to a lab so it can take a week or more to get the results and I was desperate to know. But worse still, he refused to take a sample. I needed to have missed a menstrual cycle; my *feeling* is an insufficient reason to waste taxpayer money.

—⎍⎍—

Mary's grandchild died from an ear infection. He had been taken once to his GP and twice to the accident and emergency department at the local hospital so there have been three opportunities to diagnose an ear infection in a four-year-old.

Each of them had sent him away with a case of *neurotic mother*. His high temperature resulted in a seizure which killed him. He died for the want of some antibiotics or probably even some Pamol™.

It has been traumatising for the patients, who care dearly about Mary, as do her colleagues. I attend work like some kind of zombie, numb and dumb. Finally, my period stops. I'm due to shift to the last placement before my state exams. Three months in Female Admission at Stone House. I have been a bit stretched recently. In February I started the Social Sciences: a foundation course (D102) with the Open University to try and fill my mind so there was zero time for naval gazing. It was great at first. But my latest assignment asked for my opinion of a cruel experiment where monkey babies are removed from their mothers and offered either a wire monkey mother that provided milk, or a soft cloth monkey mother that didn't. The poor monkeys clung to the soft mothers. I had written to the best of my ability (I have English language and English literature O-level with decent grades), and I had backed it all up with references – so how can they say it is wrong and strike it all out with red ink? How can my opinion be wrong? It upset me a lot, and the summer school course at Loughborough University is coming up. I intend to say what I think! I have my nursing state finals in November and the Open University exams in December. The Ward Sister on Female Admission is amazing, and I know she will help me and hassle me, and make sure I pass. I'm not sure how sympathetic she will be about the OU paper though!

—ᐱᐱᐱ—

On the ward things still need to be done. We have a middle-aged woman taking her clothes off and getting into bed with anyone. She is – or was – a missionary. Her family had been in Tanzania for years, but then her daughter got pregnant. It isn't clear to whom. She had an abortion which resulted in a psychotic breakdown for her mother. The local mental health system in Tanzania is mostly custodial since urbanisation has resulted in the loss of traditional village care systems, yet the country doesn't have the infrastructure for meaningful mental health care. There are two psychiatrists in the whole country, five assistant medical officers with some training in clinical psychiatry, and forty mental health nurses. Tanzania is a huge country, almost four times the size of the UK but only twenty million people. Returning to the UK was the only realistic thing the family could do, but the whole family is suffering. I have concerns for the daughter who is grieving for her aborted child and shoulders the burden of guilt for the state of her mother. Her mother is so seriously ill – no one is watching the daughter.

In this mixed unit our patient is getting into bed with both men and women and frightening them all. Some, though, could take advantage of her – she is slim and pretty, and doesn't look her age. Her husband is an Anglican priest and totally out of his depth. There is another daughter, younger, who has lived in Africa for almost all her life and is finding it hard to adjust to life on the edge of London. We are one down because Mary is off, and another person down because someone must stay with our bed-hopper. The ward is full and extra staff unheard of!

There are also a couple of other patients needing a close eye. One, a twenty-one-year-old guy, drinks fifteen to twenty bottles of beer a night! No one I know can even do this for one night let alone every night. He is depressed, not something many guys are admitted for. He didn't mention his drinking initially. This is a big mistake and a tip for anyone entering hospital for *any* reason; if you drink regularly then don't say you are a *just a social drinker* because you can die. This guy very nearly did. After admission and the subsequent withdrawal seizures he was sent to the emergency unit at Joyce Green where his life was saved. Now he is back. He is having injections of Ativan (i.e. lorazepam – a benzodiazepine that's quite new) to stop the delirium plus Parentrovite injections which are high-potency vitamins. He is quite big which may have helped him survive. He doesn't see himself as an alcoholic; he drinks to forget his job with British Rail. Until very recently he was an early riser, ready for work; now he can barely get out of bed at all. His job involves clearing the track, including after suicides. Probably jumpers should think about other people before they take a leap off the platform.

Then there is Jasmine. A very young girl, admitted for depression. It is uncommon for sixteen-year-olds to be admitted, though having seen twelve-year-old mothers I can see good reason for locking up some young girls. Of course she isn't locked up. Mabledon has open doors – no one is here against their will. But Jasmine has made a classic mistake amongst young girls and taken an overdose of paracetamol during the night. Not everyone understands how dangerous this is because you can buy the stuff so easily. The effect depends, of course, on body weight, state of liver etc.

Jasmine is young and fit, but tiny. She had a pack of twenty-five tablets, and fortunately she vomited at least some of them up, drawing the attention of the nightshift who found her. As few as fifteen might have been enough. Paracetamol won't kill anybody right away. If untreated; you don't feel anything and maybe think the suicide bid has failed. You might keep quiet, feeling a bit sheepish. A few days later you start to feel nauseous, and your skin may gain a yellow glow as jaundice sets in. You could start bleeding internally, dying horribly from liver failure by the end of the week. Even if you fess up to what you have done, you won't reach the top of the liver transplant list before you die. I recall a psychiatrist saying the new liver would have to be a happy organ. By now I have seen the result of enough suicides to know that it says to the family *you are not sufficient for me to want to live.* If you have children, it tells them they are not enough. Does it affect them? You bet it does!

The cut and thrust of the admission units and the hope and expectation of seeing someone leave is more exciting than simply making someone's daily life better while knowing they are not going to magically come right. What is right anyway? But along with being exciting, admission units are exhausting and stressful, lunchtime doesn't come on time (or at all), and you see stuff you wish you never had. I'm still not sure this is going to pan out for me in the long term.

I have largely given up turning up to class in the two weeks of school we get between placements. I stopped over the winter since the fire in the library was so inviting. It isn't the study that bothers me – in fact I enjoy the academic side of things, and I like the active side of things too – but I have a problem with hierarchy, and (not new to me at all) of physically sitting in a class with other people. Much like school, I find I want to kill my classmates. I wouldn't, of course, but it makes me constantly irritated. I still turn up, just not to class, unless there is a guest speaker; I pick and choose. It is odd being in a class of four, plus Terry (for now) and other oddballs. I think anyone who's missed out a section, failed one or had other problems ends up being dumped with us. When there is a guest speaker the room is packed! I have no idea who all these people are.

Today our guest speaker is a psychologist. I *am* interested, but I can't take him seriously. He looks like Rowan Atkinson from *Not the Nine O' Clock News*. Worse still he has the same mild speech impediment. It renders me silly, and it takes all my effort to stop sliding off my chair in a fit of giggles. So much for learning. I still have no idea what life as a psychologist might be like even though it is something I fancied... at least until I learned about the wire monkeys.

Drunken or Haire-Brained

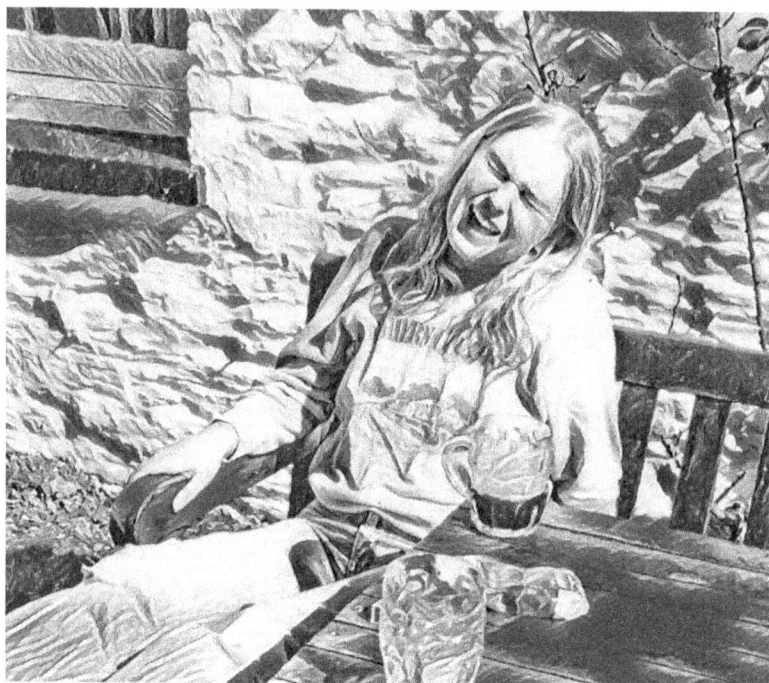

Personal photograph 1982 reimagined by lunapic.com

Chapter 14: Drunken or Haire-Brained

The teaching assessment is the only one I have left to complete. The younger and hilarious Ward Sister is keen I should pass because she has managed to garner a reputation for failing people. To be fair, one of those was my friend who became psychotic after claiming someone put marijuana in her tobacco tin. She tried to return to nursing after being sectioned under the Act to another hospital, but it quickly became clear that wasn't possible. The advice she was given was to find work in a library – somewhere quiet, more restful. Essentially her world has been turned upside down, her dreams crushed. I have no idea whether the tobacco tin claim is true, but it has wrecked her relationship, she doesn't have anywhere to live and she is currently jobless.

Losing her has also turned out to be a problem for me. I was going to teach her and the sassy little pupil nurse (who has also failed an assessment on this ward) about the difference between reactive and endogenous depression. My psychotic friend would have asked intelligent questions that would have made it easier for me to demonstrate my boundless wealth of knowledge. The pupil nurse only has boys on her mind and won't ask any questions, intelligent or otherwise, and I don't have anyone else I can take hostage. On a whole other level, this means two students have gone mad on Female Admission.

I like Stone House despite the obvious decrepitude of the building. I'm thrilled that most of the building and St Luke's chapel are now Grade II listed. This means the property is important and considered of more than special interest. The chapel isn't part of the building and was built in 1887 after the Commissioners of Lunacy decreed chapels in asylums must be detached from the main hospital buildings. I have no idea why. The old chapel was transformed into a recreation room complete with a stage and has since been turned into a dining room. There is also a clock tower, belfry and magnificent water tower that will also be saved. Apart from the tatty add-on hospital wards, the rooms have high ceilings – ten feet for the most part, but some fifteen or even twenty – and massive windows reaching from around waistline level almost to the ceiling. The windows are made of small panes but let in loads of light. I couldn't be depressed in a place like this. I'm looking forward to taking the ladies who think they have clinical depression around the trim-trail at least once a day, regardless of my shift. The fresh air helps with my overwhelming nausea and since I'm still free of bone pain, I can enjoy the trail and demonstrate the exercises.

There is something on my mind though. At night I can hear Morse code. I know how this sounds but honestly, it starts up at about 10:30 and goes on sometimes for hours. Our house was described as "semi-detached" by the estate agent. However, there are three of us in the block, so the middle house can only be described as terraced, making ours end of terrace. Middle house guy is a fireman, and we can hear his phone calls through the thin brick walls. He claims he is NOT the source of the Morse code. I don't believe I would be able to hear it from the house on the other end and I don't really want to go and ask them. She has had it tough. Her mother has been a regular inpatient at all the local hospitals, with anxiety so severe her husband left, and she literally can't do anything aside from wringing her hands. I couldn't live with her, but the daughter took her in and very recently the woman has had a leucotomy, they call it a lobotomy in the US, they are the same thing.

This is a seriously unusual and very last resort to improve her life. Banned in many countries, there are two types as far as I am aware: a prefrontal leucotomy where a piece of skull is removed or drilled into, and a transorbital leucotomy where a pick goes through the back of the eye socket to access the brain. In either case the point is to sever some connections between lobes. I have no idea which one my neighbour's mother had, but she is definitely improved for it. Overnight though, things have become much worse in their household – my neighbour's newborn baby died from cot death. It is generally believed parents are somehow to blame when babies die unexpectedly in their sleep. Something they did, or didn't do, accidental smothering with bedclothes right through to infanticide. This sounds unlikely to me.[2]

There is some interest in investigating these deaths scientifically because there are far too many for a modern country like Britain. The estimate is four or five a day and one of the suggestions I have heard regarding the cause is the rise in electro-magnetic radiation.

—⋀⋀—

I'm standing by the empty food trolley in the dining room waiting to put the dirty plates back in. I am horrendously nauseous, and I have a shot of what I can only describe as heat running down my spine and flooding my pelvis. One of the women walks towards me with a pile of plates; they look heavy, I hold out both hands and collapse.

I find myself lying on one of the hospital beds with my feet propped up on a pile of pillows. My blood pressure took a dive, and I hit the floor. The patient tells me she saw the colour drain from my face as she was holding out the plates and decided to hang onto them. Then… my period starts.

I have lost a lot of weight. I'm living on thin slices of apple – it's about all I can eat. I go back to my GP. I tell him I *am* pregnant. Then comes the problem… "When was your last period?" He gives me the sad case look, but then his face softens.

"Okay," he says, "I have a new rapid test. Put us both out of your misery."

I sit patiently in the waiting room. Then the receptionist motions me to go back in.

"Negative." He looks up to gauge my reaction, "I'm sure you will feel better once you get used to it."

---

[2] It is now known that babies should sleep on their backs. Between the first recorded "sudden infant death" in 1970 until a health campaign in Britain in 1991 around 10,000 babies would have been saved had front sleeping, first suggested by the famous Dr. Spock in 1943, been avoided.

I go home devastated. So *I am* just a sad case – pregnant in my head only. I stare at my flat chest. Confirmation.

Ironic really since the first time Stan clapped eyes on me, I was pregnant. Not long turned sixteen, he had turned up outside my house with Connor who I met on an improbable school cruise and another mate, all on big motorbikes. I thought Stan was a policeman – his bike looked distinctly like a police motorbike with a big white fairing. I didn't take much notice. I was wearing a long cheesecloth dress, stripey with ten thousand buttons down the front, a running-through-poppy-fields kind of dress. I knew I was pregnant, about twelve weeks, but I was thin enough for it not to show. I didn't much notice him (thinking he was the *fuzz*) but he noticed me.

We haven't been to the pub for a while. We used to go every night because it's cheaper to walk there, buy two pints and sip them all evening, than it is to heat the house. We have a hopeless heating system. Bricks are heated up overnight whilst electricity is cheaper and then it lets the heat out all during the day. Which is great if you are there. We both work shifts so sometimes one or even both of us benefit from it but most of the time we are both out while the house is heated and in the evening the bricks are already cold. You can have heating directly, but it costs a fortune and we simply can't afford it so it is better to take ourselves to the pub. Since it has been summer whilst I have imagined myself pregnant and therefor avoiding alcohol – we have been quite happy messing about at home.

The evenings are cooling off now and I fully intend to drown my sorrows. The Staff of Life is a mile and two tenths of country lane and a very pleasant walk, slightly uphill, which makes coming back so much the better. We are miserable, trying to make the best of it and cheer ourselves up with a bit of bat-and-trap, and we both drink too much. Stan is quietly drowning his own sorrows – we only really have each other.

Bat-and-trap is a Kentish pub game that neither of us are any good at. Usually it's a team game. The batter hits one side of a wooden seesaw that has a ball on the other end and then

114

they whack the ball as it flies up and try to get it between two posts. If the other team catches it, the batter is out. If they don't catch the ball on the fly they still have a chance to get the batter out by bowling the ball and knocking down a little door at the front of the seesaw box. We muck about in the pub garden until it's too dark to see.

I'm not much of a drinker; generally I will drink real ale – warm, cloudy, lumpy beer I can sieve through my teeth – but tonight I have Guinness. Guinness contains folate and iron. Both are good for pregnancy, but I know very well it also contains alcohol, which is not. It doesn't matter, I have proof that I am sad rather than pregnant. Four pints of Guinness is equal to ten standard drinks, so we practically roll home, and, in the morning I suffer for it. As a trooper, I still make it to work!

Funnily enough, I'm feeling pretty good. The nausea has subsided and the bone pain has stayed away. My hair is glossy, my skin is good, and I have a spring in my step. I continue with the trim trail ladies. My colleagues are happy to have a willing volunteer. I also have the second of the small chairs to finish at occupational therapy – the first one I completed so long ago I have probably forgotten how to do it. I might as well have something to remember my stay. I try not to dwell on the lack of pregnancy, but I cannot help noticing there are loads of baby-oriented ads on the TV and almost everyone I see is pushing a pram. My chairs might not ever be needed.

We decide to take the wall out between the toilet and bathroom and move it downstairs (the wall not the toilet), to separate the hall from the lounge and reuse the old toilet door to enter the lounge from the hallway, it looks great and cost us next to nothing. I can't drink coffee or alcohol – the smell of either is wrong. What I do want is German cheesecake which is hard to get, not cheap, and fattening. My belly is already getting a pot!

I'm off to Loughborough for summer school in less than two weeks. I haven't been away from Stan for more than a couple of days since we married, though last year he did leave me home alone when he went to Norwich University for his course T101 Living with Technology. He had a great time. I went with him to drop him off and we met the "TADpoles". TAD292 are Art and Environment students. They have a reputation for doing mad things and they certainly entertained everyone on arrival. I am so looking forward to Loughborough. The timing is good because my period will have finished by the time I go – hours on a bus is no fun anyway, but with my period it would be worse.

Except... it doesn't come.

Is it delayed by the stress of having so much to do, the stress of the failed pregnancy, or perhaps weight loss (though that seems to be rapidly reversing)? Please don't let me be pregnant after drinking four pints of Guinness.

The GP looks up at me and rolls his eyes. I know what he is thinking.

"Please," I tell him, "my period is late, I have to go to Loughborough, and I drank four pints of Guinness when you told me I wasn't pregnant. You *have* to do a test."

He agrees. I wait.

My GP is all smiles and heartily congratulates me. How relieved I must be to have a positive test at last.

I want the earth to swallow me up – how can history repeat? Maybe I wasn't pregnant at the time of the Guinness fest, though we hadn't stopped practising. After all, I had a negative test.

The receptionist organises an appointment, and I tell her I want to go to Gravesend rather than All Saints for my care. All Saints was originally a workhouse, it should have closed decades ago. The clinic at Gravesend is more modern and less daunting, it means something to have a choice. Gravesend clinic can squash me in before I go to Loughborough. I have a heap of questions.

In France and Italy some mothers are advised to start drinking wine (if they didn't already) to take the edge off morning sickness. The drug containing thalidomide was supposed to be a safe way to avoid morning sickness too. My mum was offered it but fortunately turned it down. I think the boy with half an arm who used to hit me on the SS *Fairstar* when we emigrated to Australia was probably afflicted (mildly) by thalidomide. The notion that alcohol can cause problems hasn't hit mainstream, but as an avid reader of the *New Scientist*, since I spent my schooldays holed up in the library rather than in class, I do have some knowledge about it.

In fact, the link between alcohol and pregnancy can be dated back a long way. Aristotle's *Problemata:*

Foolish, drunken, or haire-brain women most often bring forth children like unto themselves, morose and languid.

I don't consider myself foolish, drunken or haire-brained. I wish I'd never had the negative test because I had already stopped drinking to increase my chances of a perfect child. I'm not sure I could cope with a disabled child. My meticulous planning has gone awry. Before I slash my wrists, I need the advice of the Chief Obstetrician.

This proves more problematic than I thought. The Junior Doctor at the clinic informs me I am at least 14 weeks pregnant, and it seems the top Doctor only sees problem pregnancies. If two full-blown periods, a negative test and four pints of Guinness is not a problem then what is? I refuse to leave until I see him, and they make me wait for hours.

When he arrives he has little patience for me. I explain how distressed I am, evidenced by tears – but he is totally dismissive. One night of alcohol after the first trimester is hardly worthy of wasting his time – and more to the point, if I was a responsible adult I should have been at the clinic sooner. I tried to explain the refused test, the negative test, but he walked away saying I had better attend future appointments and don't be surprised if I end up with a caesarean because of pelvic insufficiency – it looks like I have a big baby.

Initially I am reassured. The top doctor has bigger problems than me. He doesn't think one night of alcohol is an issue. Either he doesn't get it or doesn't care. But then I start thinking what else *could* he say to someone already fragile? "You are an idiot, foolish and haire-brained, and have done untold damage." What would be the point?

-\/\/\-

While I have been rostered off a suicidal woman was admitted. She is dead already. She was placed into one of the seclusion rooms. There are two identical rooms with high ceilings and huge windows. Each window has thirty panes of glass. With a footprint similar to single bedroom in a modern house, the rooms are higher than they are wide. Each has a radiator, tiny basin and nothing else. Most of the rooms in the hospital, and even the corridors, are plastered or have wooden panels; these have brick, whitewashed walls. From the windowsill down to the floor they are painted, one a dark pink and the other a sort of turquoise. Each room has a colour matched flowery frieze between the coloured bottom and whitewashed top. The light is so good it would delight an artist but clearly this lady was seriously unhappy.

The mattress on the floor has sheet, blanket and bedcover, machine stitched together in one-inch squares. It is impossible to rip and there isn't anything to hang yourself on. Without a weapon tougher than a toothbrush there is no way of smashing the toughened glass. Yet she is dead. She worked her toothpaste tube back and forth until she could rip it. Since it's made of metal, she was then able to slash her wrists with the ragged edge and bled to death before anyone checked on her. How long would it have taken? The checks should have been every fifteen minutes. I don't know if they were. Apparently the blood was everywhere; she wouldn't have lasted long.

As I am pregnant, and we don't have a car, we have been looking out for one. We spotted the metallic turquoise Volkswagen Beetle parked on a slope on the concrete in front of the local dealer's showroom. Our neighbour has a Beetle and has always been happy with it. It might even fit in our garage, though then you probably couldn't open the doors to get out and climbing out the back door and over the engine would be difficult. She is pretty.

118

Chapter 15: Alternate Education

There are a few of us Open University students on the coach from London. The van driver collecting us from Loughborough coach station has bad news.

"There have been two rapes on campus, so no one will be allowed out after dark, and security guards will be walking you to and from the accommodation."

We look at him in disbelief and then at each other. Some of them look pretty pissed off and I realise not everyone is here solely for their education. I had intended to study flat tack and sort out the red ink and wire monkey problem rather than hit the night clubs. We search through bags disgorged from the coach to find ours and start loading them into the trailer hooked onto the minivan.

One of the girls on the course is clearly pregnant; I congratulate her and tell her that I, too, am full of arms and legs! We are both about sixteen weeks and one of the boys asks quite pointedly of my new friend, "How come you're fat and she has no belly at all?" He looks at me as if I'm lying.

I do have a slight belly, but I already feel enough like an imposter – she has quite a bump.

"Third baby," she says. "All my muscles have gone to pot."
I don't like the sound of that!

"Have you made sure they put you near the loo?" she asks.
"I got a first-floor room next to the bathroom."

"I didn't even think of it, but bugger, let's hope I am close because it will be a disaster at night if I'm not." She is clearly more experienced than I am.

We clamber into the minivan, and once at the university digs, I find I'm on the top floor and as far from the loo as you can get... shit. I don't know if I can ask for a change. I don't want to make a fuss, so I unpack. We are meeting soon for an initial session which isn't really part of the course but is to help with the research for a project needed by a student who's far ahead of my first-year status.

In a darkened lecture theatre, our job is to look at a series of slides and determine how manly each picture is. A lot of them are neither manly nor unmanly – a bloke driving a car, standing in a lift. I guess that's to even out those scoring too high or too low? Some of the pictures are yuk. Body builders with oiled skin over muscles and veins – how can anyone like that kind of thing? They're probably pumped full of steroids, and infertile. I judge the picture of Daley Thompson holding the tiniest baby as the manliest of all. Daley Thompson is a superhero of mine. I'm not prone to superheroes; you must be quite special to get on my list! He won the gold medal in the 1980 Olympics. Unfortunately 66 countries boycotted the games because of the Soviet–Afghan War. It is never satisfactory when you are not competing against the whole world, and I'm still not sure why the UK didn't boycott those games. The team simply didn't march at the opening ceremony; their Chef-de-Mission carried the flag. A bit limp in terms of protest. However, Daley has broken the world record for the decathlon twice, which cements his dominance in my eyes. The photo topping my poll wasn't because it showed him – it could have been anyone – but because of his muscular body providing safety for a vulnerable baby.

Chatting with the other students, we find the girls mostly went for the Daley Thompson photo. A few others went for Daley drinking orange juice which I had put second. The boys in the group went for the bodybuilder or beer-slugging types. What is wrong with them? The way guys think is a mystery to me. When I had my first motorbike, I would be regularly taking other people's girlfriends home at the end of their evening date. Funnily enough they preferred the safe and sedate ride they got on the back of my bike rather than having the pants scared off them by their boyfriends' riding. Demonstrating what a dick you are does not impress girls. These male friends of mine aren't idiots and yet the temptation to show off was clearly too great.

Our security guards escort us to the dining room. This is unnerving and a lot of the others were looking forward to sampling the delights of Loughborough. In fact, I have been here before. My close friend – drop-dead gorgeous Rick – was at university here. I stayed with him, we went to concerts together, we dropped acid together and I never jumped his bones because it is the best way of destroying a great friendship. Although I made an exception for Stan!

Escorted back to the accommodation block, I find the day's travels have caught up with me and I am exhausted. After a warm shower and trying to slink back along the corridor wrapped in a towel, I realise it is going to be torture doing this a couple of times (at least) during the night. Rummaging through the cupboards, I find a saucepan. Not very big, but then how much can one person pee overnight?

Quite a bit, is the answer. I look at the pot in the cold light of day. The room doesn't have a sink, and I can't leave it there in the heat of the dying days of summer, but if I try carrying it the length of the corridor it will definitely spill. The window is my only hope; if I chuck it out I won't be seen. The window faces a forested area, and the chances of anyone happening to be hanging out of their window this early in the morning are zero.

Some pee slips out as I get the pot balanced on the windowsill; never mind, I can mop it up. I ease the window open. It is one of those metal windows with green, flaky paint. I can fix it wide open with the long metal lever. With both hands free to tilt the pot, and trying not to spill more, I tip it out. There is a yell from below. I slam the window shut as quickly as I can.

As we are escorted to breakfast it has spread amongst the students that one of the security guards got soaked from above this morning whilst doing his rounds. It is a complete mystery. Ordinarily I would crack up. I force a smile; he can easily identify the likely occupants on each floor. I don't think they realise it was urine.

The course D102 covers psychology, sociology, economics and politics. I had thought taking psychology would help me grow as a nurse; the other subjects are a requirement of the course. Economics is more interesting than I expected and even politics isn't as dull as it sounds. Psychology might make me a better person, but I can see it isn't for me. If you don't agree with the opinion of the lecturer, then you are wrong. I was born a rebel, and I can't fit in.

You must take two foundation courses out of five. I will pass D102 because I paid for it and I won't waste money. A soft option for next year would be Living with Technology (T101), because Stan has already done it and, let's be honest, I had my sticky beak into it all the time. It wouldn't be much of a challenge though and the idea is to fill my mind all of the time. I have also heard that babies can make you lose any brains you may have had. M101 is maths and therefor out – which leaves arts (A101) or sciences (S101). I have always been interested in science – I spent vast tracts of my time in the school library reading about famous scientists – but I failed chemistry more dismally than anyone at my school ever has! Problem is, I don't have any skills in the arts either. I was told music wasn't an option for me (when everyone else got to choose between art and music) but I'm hopeless at art as well. I was keen enough to audition for A Midsummer Night's Dream at school and I got the part of Mustardseed, a fairy in the court of Titania. I had to crawl out from under the stage and my only line was "Mustardseed." I'd wanted the part of Puck, Oberon's mischievous sidekick – totally the part for me – but given my lack of talent I was lucky to get on stage at all.

My heart isn't in the Open University course work though, sociology bores me, psychology annoys me and there is no point in politics. My plans for a degree in psychology have gone off the rails and I'm not getting much out of this block course. Apart from being under guard and in fear of a rapist, I'm struggling to remain interested, and no one cares what I think about the red ink. The baby monkeys and wire mothers still play on my mind.

At lunchtime we are free of the guards if we stick to the central areas of the dining room and quad. I am stretched out in the sun on a handily placed boulder, an older lady close by, and I can't help but notice she has her nose buried in a science book. "I would love to do science," I tell her, "but I am too stupid."

She looks up and smiles. "It isn't about how smart you are, but about how badly you want it. How hard are you prepared to try?"

She goes on to tell me that every time there is a zero on the end of her birthday she takes up something new. At sixty she took up a degree in science. I like this woman immediately and I love the new things idea. It is quite a while until there is a zero at the end of my birthday, but I will keep it in mind. She explains that since I must take two foundation courses and I will already have D102, how about I take Science (S101) next year, and then I can enrol the following year for the second level course Biology Brain and Behaviour (SD286), which is psychology from a scientific slant. I might find it more interesting.

This little encounter has boosted my enthusiasm.

I find things feel resolved in my head. I ensure I don't overfill the saucepan during the night, and between pees I hatch another plan. On TV I watched a travel show where they had a meal in a Pullman coach on a train on the North Yorkshire Moor. Stan has long banged on about the trainset he had as a boy which had a Pullman coach. He doesn't know there is a Christmas trainset, with said coach, under our bed! But what if we could travel on the actual coach? It isn't the sort of thing you can do with a baby in tow.

Autumn isn't ideal to be on the moor, but we have the autumn term break coming up. Probably our last chance. It is a long way to drive, and I would have to drive all the way, but maybe he could get his car licence before then. He needs to get it anyway – how can he rush me to the hospital when the baby comes on the back of his bike?

—∿—

Back on Female Admission after my stint as a uni student I am happier. My health is great, I have a plan for my studies, a revision plan for my State Finals and a plan for a holiday. I am pregnant, despite the faffing about, and the timing isn't great, but I will have finished the qualification long before the baby is due.

There is a bit of excitement: the nurses have been taking strike action. Not only the nurses, to be fair, but all sorts of health workers after rejecting a 5% pay offer. Health workers' wages are poor, and the good nature of people means the word *vocation* is used to pretend people don't mind being poorly paid. Students are not allowed to be involved in strike action, but today 22nd of September (1982) the TUC (Trades Union Congress) have organised a day of action by health workers, and sympathetic action by other unions. The nurses on Female Geriatrics made placards, helped by some of the patients, and the patients are lined up on the picket line. I go and visit them; they are having a ball waving placards and yelling. No one wants to cross the picket line because people are generally in agreement – hospital workers should have more pay. But any potential scabs wouldn't have wanted to face the ladies from Female Geriatrics anyway, especially old Ma Cummings, who will defend the nurses to her death!

The teaching assessment goes as well as it could. The pupil nurse didn't ask any questions, but Sister dragged everything I know out of me. The only criticism she has is that since there was a desk between me and my audience (two people) I seemed unnecessarily distant. I'll take that; it's still a pass. So – I have passed all my assessments at the first attempt and all my assignments.

The truth is I have spent large swathes of the school time in the library. I started with good intentions and at first it wasn't so bad. There was a fair amount of discussion with the Mauritian boys there, but the class is too small; Mike and I are the only ones with anything to say. I became bored long ago. The assignments have basically been case studies, so I knocked out as many as I could – it is interesting and a good way to learn. When anyone came searching for me, I could flick through my pile and find something vaguely suitable. It never failed.

A friend of Stan's came for the weekend. He is a bit of a geek and tends to stand a bit too close which seems creepy, but he's smart. Walking back from the pub, I bemoaned the fact that the Morse code would likely start as soon as we got back. He declared that he would get to the bottom of it. I was a bit cheered that he even believed me. He has a ham radio set up in his car. He found the Morse code emitter almost immediately. It is a guy just around the corner; he starts up as soon as he gets home from the pub. Very likely it is the same pub!

Even though I could be the sober driver, we prefer to walk to and from the pub. The walk is surreal in the silence, the overhanging trees making almost a tunnel to walk through. Especially in the snow it is like an enchanted garden. One night Stan and I saw lights in the sky that rose straight up from behind the houses and trees in the direction of the Medway River, then disappeared. They reappeared shortly after and lowered to the ground in a straight line, all in total silence. We vowed never to speak of it. Until we found from the local newspaper that the Harrier jump jets had been practising night manoeuvres from the local base.

Most people drive to the pub since the chances of getting busted for drink driving are virtually zero here. Morse code guy must drive to have started before I get home, and he has offered to pack it in. I say if he lets me fall asleep first it probably won't wake me up. Knowing what it is now, I can probably ignore it.

My period starts a few days before our holiday. I have no idea what to think – I should be about nineteen weeks pregnant. I feel pregnant, but I'm not certain I have felt any movements. Reluctantly, I front up to my GP, but his demeanour is much improved from my previous visits. He manages to pick up a heartbeat with his stethoscope and he reassures me yes, my pregnancy is atypical, but I should trust my own feelings. That's a bit of a change of position!

What better way to learn to drive than a long journey with varied terrain and an unknown destination? What could possibly go wrong?

The brakes seize by Milton Keynes and Stan does roadside repairs. By the time we reach the North Yorkshire moors the brakes are the least of our problems, and the car limps into the carpark of the Mallyan Hotel. Then the local garage sets it alight! The garage owner assures us there isn't a problem, just a blown light bulb. This can't be true and they admit to a small fire in the carburettor. We pay and don't discuss the fire.

The pinnacle of the trip and the answer to Stan's question, "Why am I taking my wedding suit on holiday?" is on our last day. I'm wearing my soft grey velvet dress, probably for the last time, and his suit matches it perfectly (entirely unplanned). We aren't too cold as we wait on the station a short walk from the hotel and catch the train to Grosmont. The steam train leaves from Grosmont, goes to Pickering (through Goathland where we are staying) and returns to Grosmont, we can get off at Goathland Station on the way back and not lose much of our trip. In total it is about thirty-five miles that we will be on the train.

Because it is so late in the year we won't see much of the scenery. The carriage is the reason to be here which is just as well, because we have barely moved away from the station when the train stops. It starts and stops a few more times and then the steward comes through the carriages with complimentary wine, which of course I don't drink, but it is to soothe a problem. The power is off. This is a steam train with gas lighting... and an electric galley.

We are seated four to a table, and fortunately the couple sharing our table are good fun. We have plenty to talk about and we don't notice darkness falling until we realise we can't see. The train moves and it seems the gas lighting is only for show – electric lights are needed to see well enough to eat your dinner... if there was any. The steward is fabulous and brings candles, more wine, but not dinner.

126

In my head I see Basil Fawlty on his way to get duck from his mate Andre's restaurant after new chef Kurt (gay and alcoholic) gets overly drunk after being rejected by Manuel. I don't think this scenario is quite like that, but I am wondering where our meals are coming from.

Eventually we have a great night in the half-light and the meals are fantastic. Stan is super happy with the treat, the train, the meal and the company, and the outages mean the merriment goes on for longer than anticipated. We get dropped at Goathland Station and wobble back to the hotel – him tipsy, me exhausted.

–◡◠–

All I have to do is study for the finals and work my shifts until the end of the year. In a couple of weeks we have the birthday of our friend's daughter. She is one, but she has recently been diagnosed with a brain tumour and isn't expected to make her second birthday. I feel self-conscious, being pregnant, but I'm not counting any chickens yet. I'm twenty-one weeks, and I've had a hard time trying to convince anyone of it. Aside from the negative pregnancy tests, I have lost a lot of weight due to vomiting so my bump barely shows, but I need a new bra – immediately.

127

The Short-Lived Beetle

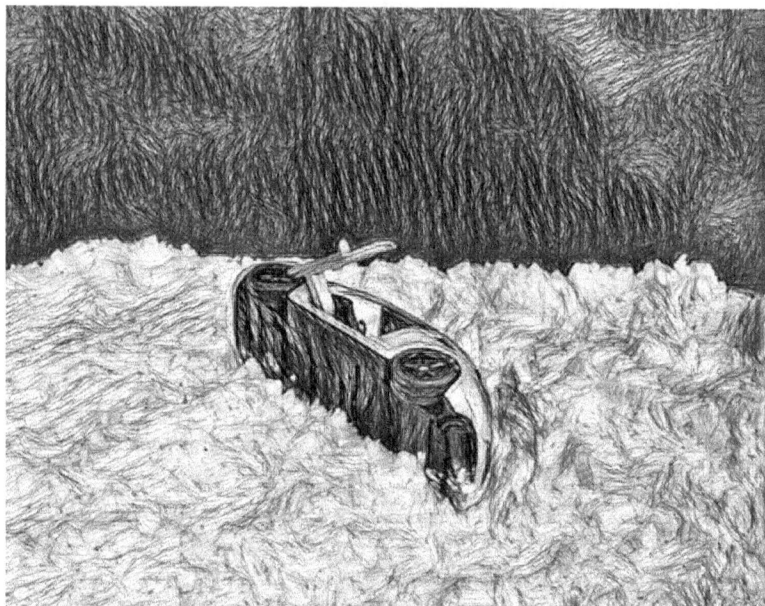

Photograph of reenactment; toy car in a tray of flour and reimagined by lunapic.com

Chapter 16: Crashing Out

I hit ice, but I have a plan. I aim the sliding car toward a field I know has been recently ploughed; I imagine it will slow the car, which will stop in the soft furrows buried beneath the snow. But I hit an inconveniently placed power-pole. There is a dreadful crack and my dear little Beetle rolls.

I find myself held awkwardly sideways by the seatbelt, the driver's door pinned by the furrows of the field, and without the strength to undo the seatbelt – I'm stuck. I can't climb up and haul myself out of the hole where there used to be a passenger door even if I could manage to undo the seat belt. In those few terrifying minutes Stan has disappeared. Could I have been out cold for a few seconds? A few minutes? Where the hell has Stan gone?

It's worse than that – I am dead. A bright light blinds my eyes, and an astronaut reaches into the car from the clear, starry sky visible through the passenger door opening. He is massively strong; I say he because of the smell – leather and grease. Holding my weight with one arm and grappling with the seatbelt with the other, he pulls me from the car in a single haul and lays me on the snow-covered field.

"Is there a blanket in the car?" he asks.

I hadn't imagined dialogue after death.

Then the sky pulses with blue flashing lights. I don't believe in the afterlife, and I never pictured it as a freezing outdoor disco.

A cheery, tubby ambo officer is "live" on the ploughed field, and I'm confused. The astronaut pulls off his helmet and starts talking to the ambo. "Yes, I pulled her out. No, there was no one else in the car."

Now I have to liven up. "Stan! Stanleeeey!"

The ambulance officer comes over. "What's up, love?"

"My husband, Stan – he was in the car. I don't know where he went."

The astronaut assures ambo man there wasn't anyone else, so I have to up the ante and I get seriously loud.

129

"Stanleeeey!" My shrill echoes in the dark.

Then we all notice the lean on the power-pole.

"Hell – we gotta get you out of here, love."

I dig my heels in – he was in the car, and I am not going anywhere until he is found. Clearly I can't stay on the snow under a power-pole about to topple. Another ambulance officer takes over, the astronaut disappears amidst the unmistakable roar of a motorbike, and the chubby guy goes into the darkness with a flashlight. Eventually rounding up my sweetheart, who is looking for something but has forgotten what.

They are taking us to the Medway Maritime Hospital. This was originally a naval hospital built in 1905, but it has a modern A&E department; we should be good. I tell the ambos I'm pregnant; they are more concerned about Stan who isn't making sense and has a nasty bang on the right side of his head. I have moderate bangs on both sides, but they think he is worse.

At the hospital they determine he was driving because the bang is on the right side of his head, sustained when the car rolled. He doesn't know whether he was driving or not, but I do. Firstly, I am the one with the licence, and since I'm pregnant I'm also the sober driver. I hit ice and wound up destroying a power-pole.

They reckon the bang would be on the left if he were the passenger. They want to keep him and send me to All Saints where they have a baby unit. The same All Saints that I didn't want to be referred to for my pregnancy. It was declared unfit to be a hospital more than a decade ago. But, since I now have abdominal pain, and we are in the wrong area, All Saints is my only hope.

Stan won't have a bar of being left behind, so we pile back into the ambulance; it is a bit like having a posh taxi. The streets are empty – it's the middle of the night.

A quick examination determines I am in the early stages of labour and my cervix is softening. They can't cope with a baby as premature as this. Builders are in the process of constructing a unit that could, but for now they hook up a

Ventolin drip which puts me in a state of mild panic. Matron gets on the phone. She assures us there is a plane on standby and an ambulance waiting to take me to the airport. I can see the lights of the ambulance. Not like a disco now but a reassuring steady blue pulse, comforting in a way. I imagine this is going to be a matter of a quick phone call and we will be on the road again. But it isn't like that. I can hear one side of the conversation as she runs swiftly through the details

"Twenty-three weeks, car crash, otherwise fit... oh, you're full. OK, thanks" and then again, and again, and again and still the pulsing blue light but my hopes are fading and my heart is racing as the Ventolin flows through my veins.

Eventually Matron comes back but I already know, there isn't anywhere with both the skills and the room. She rubs my back and tells me they will find a room for me rather than leave me on a busy ward. She isn't sure about Stan; he can't go home with a head injury; they get a doctor to flash a light into his eyes. They did that at Medway, he does the same to me. I have a problem with the reaction of my left pupil, Stan's main problem is with his right. It doesn't make any sense. I tell them I was driving. They don't argue but I can tell they don't believe me. The power is out to the whole of the Hoo Peninsular. My neighbours will hate me. I am not allowed to eat or drink but they fuss around Stan, making him cups of tea and jam on toast. They push together a couple of armchairs and put a blanket over him. He is out like a light. In the end, I drift off to sleep.

When I wake, Stan isn't there, but he quickly appears. "Phoned your mum," he says. The nurses are fussing over him about breakfast. I don't get any fuss. I *am* still pregnant but I spent so long being told I wasn't, then I had around eight weeks of being pregnant and being believed, and then it turns out it is all so fragile. I am stable enough to move to a ward. The nurse keeps telling me to calm down. I don't know why I'm so anxious; it isn't like me at all. The giving set for the Ventolin keeps running faster. As it speeds up, so does my heart. The nurse keeps slowing it down, but it speeds up again

131

of its own accord. I'm supposed to rest, yet how can I? Mum turns up, and I am in a real state. She says that Stan phoned to say I had been in a car crash but didn't say where. She had to phone half the hospitals in Kent looking for me.

I shouldn't have been driving. I was too tired, the roads too icy and the trip was too long so late at night. It had also been a stressful event – we'd been at the birthday party for the dying one-year-old, there to support her parents. Not only are they facing the loss of their baby before her second birthday, but both sets of grandmothers have said the child's brain tumour is the result of her having been conceived out of wedlock... God's punishment. Who is this benevolent creator that should smite a child with a brain tumour to chastise the parents for having a quickie – try before you buy is my motto.

However, the God excuse is no better than the GP who declared there was nothing wrong with the baby – just another neurotic mother having gone back to work instead of caring for her infant. Going to work and leaving your child in the capable hands of an experienced caregiver cannot result in missing milestones. If that was the case then how have babies rolled over, smiled and made noises in the absence of fathers – or don't they count for anything? Bills must be paid; a working mother should be an OK thing in the enlightened 80s, but views take a long time to change.

We should have stayed over – we could have stayed over – but I wanted my own bed. Instead, I have a hospital bed, a baby of uncertain status and very likely an entire peninsular of haters!

I'm struggling to cope with Mum. She is disturbed by seeing the state I'm in and calls the nurse, who is aghast at the speed of the giving set and slows it down. I feel – perhaps I'm paranoid – that she hints I have been speeding it up myself. Stan has gone home for a change of clothes and confirms the power pole is being replaced – on a Sunday – and I wonder who will be paying for it. No one seems worried about him now and I have had time to think about things. I know I was driving. As the car rolled, he hit the right side of his head on mine, hence the bump on his right and bumps on my right and left. Clearly my head is harder than his!

The good news is the Ventolin has stopped the labour and I can go home. The bad news – I'm on total bed rest. After three years of training my State Finals are in a couple of weeks. An event I shall miss. What a mess! At least Stan can drive, and he has scored a cheap Mini off a guy at work. He still needs a full licence holder in the car, though, so now he will have to sit his test, no excuses. The Mini is… I am not sure how best to describe it. Green with a silver roof that looks like it's been hand painted. The floor seems to move separately from the body, and we quickly discover what can only be described as "a total loss oil system", where every trip we find we must add more oil. We joke that it uses more oil than petrol – not a very funny joke obviously

My neighbour had been on bed rest. She has had a few miscarriages. She has a live baby now after spending the entire pregnancy either in bed or in hospital. I have no idea how she did it. I have a bed made up in the lounge, ants in my pants, and a TV without a remote. It has rabbit ears and barely does colour. Stan leaves me with a packed lunch, some books and the TV is on. Bed rest is, in fact, nonsense. I don't have a commode, which sees me crawling carefully up the stairs to the loo several times a day. After peeing in the saucepan at Loughborough, I'm wary of overflowing any container and risking the carpet. I can't even study for my finals. The next opportunity is March and then only if the baby has been born (should we get that far). I cannot plan so far ahead. Plus, they have told me that to be awarded the qualification I have to go back and complete the missing time. I am short on hours, which mount up to eight weeks and must be in one of the admission units. I don't get a say where and all are a long drive. I either leave the baby with a minder or forfeit the qualification.

Next week I have the planned appointment at Gravesend where I got yelled at before. I guess I must get out of bed for that! I snuggle up, using the cheap heat while knowing we will have to freeze tonight. No pub to keep us warm and no heat left in the bricks.

Chapter 17: Resting in Bed

Every day is the same, until today. Today the TV catches fire. Bed rest or not, I cannot ignore a flaming TV. I get up calmly, as the flames leap from the back and upwards against the wall that covers the side of the stairs. That is going to need scrubbing. Dragging the plug out of the socket by its lead, I drop it and walk gingerly to the kitchen to get a pan which I fill from the tap. I'm trying very hard not to panic; this is hardly bed rest. I chuck water over the TV from a distance because I cannot remember if you should put water on an electrical fire or you should not. Nothing bad happens and I suspect the TV was never going to work again whatever I did.

Since I can't go anywhere or do anything and the TV is broken, I get Stan to buy a knitting machine. They are all the rage. I can knit quite well the traditional way – I learned when I worked at the Clearing House. I recently knitted a dress and jacket in very fine turquoise cotton, not that I ever go anywhere to wear that kind of thing. Sheila, the Clearing House switchboard operator, taught me, horrified that my mother hadn't. She was using the knitting lessons as an excuse to make sure I had lunch; she knew I was poor. She always claimed to have brought too much food with her, and said it would go to waste.

Mum wasn't really a knitter… or a sewer. She had a sewing machine but since Aunt Em was a brilliant machinist it was easier to get her to do any sewing. Aunt Em would make dresses for me, and with the leftover fabric she made matching knickers. When I went on the school cruise, I hired my dresses and knickers out, ten new pence for the set for the evening (two shillings in old money, or two bob as Granddad would say). I had a bunch of nail varnishes, and I let the hirers of the dresses use those for an extra shilling. I probably didn't make much on the nail varnish, but I was bringing in 40 or 50 new pence a day most days. That was an odd thing, I never found out how I got to be on the cruise. I didn't even take the notice home because we couldn't afford it. Mum asked me about it after it was mentioned at the parent-teacher interviews. I told her I wasn't interested. That was a lie but I knew I couldn't go, so why make a fuss. Even if we could afford it, there was a draw to get in because it would be wildly oversubscribed. Something was going on because the scholarship kids outnumbered the rich kids and we cruised the Baltic for ten days. That's where I met Connor, we crawled through the disco hunting for snarks and got banned.

Point is, I had never learned to sew properly either. Stan's mum is a good machinist, but she gets me to explain patterns to her because what I am good at is interpreting written instructions, whereas she likes to be shown. I soon teach myself to use the knitting machine, it is fiddly, and I jam it up a few times, but I make a super lacy pink baby shawl. After all, I am expecting a girl – my friends all say so and the older aunties swung my wedding ring over my belly and confirmed it!

Stan, the Mini and I make it to Gravesend for the appointment. My Beetle has been towed to the garage that did the service before we went on our secret holiday. The brakes hadn't even made it halfway before they seized on, so we feel they didn't do a proper job. Then the people in Goathland fixed it and set fire to it so it might be hard to prove our case – but we are taking them to the small claims court anyway. Now the Beetle is very broken, but I'm hoping the chassis is straight and the car can be repaired. I would say it is still a better bet than this Mini, but this is what we have, and I am grateful for it.

The maternity unit at the hospital doesn't know anything about the car crash. I suppose it would be too much to hope notes might get transferred from one district to another, so I explain the whole sorry saga. They don't believe me – which is ludicrous because I have a huge seatbelt-shaped bruise across my torso plus an unreliable witness who can't remember anything! They don't think bed rest is warranted and yet don't think I should return to work. This is the worst of both worlds in terms of my qualification. I could accept its loss to save this precious baby – but if it isn't necessary then what the hell am I doing? I explain there hasn't been any movement, and some young dumb junior doctor suggests the baby's back is broken. Just the news I need. I try to dismiss it as coming from a poorly informed doctor who probably knows as much about pregnancy as I do, but I can't help hearing his voice on the journey home.

We have barely got in when there is frantic banging on the door. We used to be able to see who was at the door but with our modifications we have to go into the noticeably colder little hallway where we are right by the glass door. It is Julie from next door. She is leaving in a hurry before her husband gets back from work. She is going to stay with her sister.

She must be desperate; her sister is a lesbian. While I couldn't care less, to Julie it is a major sin that has torn the family apart. For her to be staying there she must have limited options. I had no idea there was anything wrong, but her main issue right now is her baby's crib – a Victorian affair, all lace and silk. The thing rocks and looks astonishing, but I can imagine vomit in the intricate embroidery. Anyway, it won't fit in her car. To keep it safe we manhandle it upstairs to the back bedroom.

I'm thankful I have bought a Moses basket – to do with Moses and bulrushes, and it really is just a basket. I have some cotton fabric – dusky pink squares on a white background – to make a quilt. It is double sided, so the other side is white squares on a pink background. I don't want vomit in the basket weave, so I hope I have enough fabric to line it. It will be handy for carrying the baby from room to room. I really wouldn't pay the kind of money Julie must have paid for an elaborate thing the kid won't even sleep in for long. I have heard of babies sleeping in drawers, and I remember the one on my community placement that slept in a cardboard box on top of the TV.

I don't mind helping her out. She did give us practically all her crockery when Stan and I had a dispute over the washing up. It was when he started on the appalling shift at the closer power station, it was his turn to wash the dishes and he wouldn't because he thought it was my turn. We are both a little stubborn and our dirty dishes piled up on the draining board. When we ran out we borrowed Julie's. Eventually she sheepishly knocked on the door and asked for her plates back. The stack of unwashed dishes was a health hazard by then and we had to wash up, I caved first.

Julie goes to her sister and Stan takes off on his bike for the late shift. I really do need some bed rest whether it's necessary or not. I can't sleep – the broken back comment is playing on my mind. The only useful thing to come out of this is the extra time that I can put into the Open University course. I can at least sit the exam and revise without distraction. Economics has turned out to be the most interesting part of the course – who would have predicted that! It isn't any use to me though; no way am I going back to office type work.

Bright lights are beaming into the lounge; there is a lorry outside. I must have fallen asleep because it is dark. I would have closed the curtains by now, trying to keep some warmth in as the bricks run out of heat. What *is* going on? A couple of blokes are removing the furniture from next door.

I ring the number Julie gave me. "Julie, someone is robbing your house. They have a big lorry."

"Yes," she says, "I expected something like that. It's Mark – he threatened to throw boiling water over me while I was holding Johnathon. I told him to leave."

"I think he is taking everything, Julie."

"He can have it, just don't give him that crib."

"Don't worry, I'm not even going out there. I shall draw the curtains and ignore them. I thought you should know, is all."

"Thanks. Hopefully he will have gone by tomorrow, and then I can work out what to do next."

I close the curtains while they are inside her house – and it is her house – then put the light on. I don't want to draw attention to the place. We aren't allowed fences, trees or even bushes due to line-of-sight rules. This means zero privacy. The postman walks as close to the windows as you can get, going from door to door, and so does the milkman. So close, they brush the windows as they pass. Since I was put on bed rest I've been having a row with the milkman. I won't get up at 6 a.m. when he knocks for payment and so he is refusing to deliver. It doesn't stop him walking across our garden to go from one house to the next. I wander into the kitchen, put the kettle on and search the cupboard for something to eat.

Next thing there is angry bashing at the front door. "Give me the crib. I know that bitch has left it!"

"I have no idea what you're talking about," I lie. "Leave me alone – you know I'm on bed rest."

I slump onto the bottom step of the staircase. He can see well enough through the patterned glass to know I am there, but I want to be close to the phone in case he doesn't leave.

His aggression is escalating. The door is rattling with his thumps and my pulse is rising with it.

"Just give it to me. I'm going to kick this glass in and take it anyway."

Right, that is a threat; I ring the police. I don't think he realises I'm on the phone because he's making such a racket, and you can't see through the glass well enough to see what is going on – walling the lounge off has made the hallway dark.

"I have a man banging on my door threatening to break it down – I am pregnant and scared."

They tell me they can only do something if he actually breaks in.

I can't believe my ears. I know it would take them at least twenty minutes from the cop shop, even with lights and sirens. It crosses my mind to tell them not to worry because I have a gun. I don't, of course – the implied threat might backfire, and I could end up in trouble. I slam down the phone in disgust, why do I pay rates and tax? But the glass must be tougher than average – he has been kicking it hard enough I would have expected it to smash – it looks like the wooden frame might give way first.

Then his mate yells, "Leave it. Let's get out of here."

Mark turns, and in a flash the lorry is gone.

139

I sit on the step and burst into tears.

Julie returns the next day and we go together to inspect the house. Everything that could be removed has gone. He has taken the toilet roll and the holder and all the light fittings. She is incredibly stoic and arranges to get the locks changed. I lend her some crockery and our camping stove.

I don't know why she married him. He's quite a bit younger and I think he thought he was onto a good thing, not many women own their own home.

Mind you, it took Stan long enough to fall for me. Although he had noticed me when I was sixteen, he had sensed I was with Connor which I wasn't. Even after we became friends, he viewed me as a sister at best, and mostly as a nuisance.

It wasn't until the summer of 1977, three of us, me Stan and Mick went to the TT (Tourist Trophy) races in the Isle of Man. We were booked into a hotel along the promenade, in Douglas – not in the centre of town but certainly walking distance. We left from Essex and rode through the night to be in time for the Liverpool ferry. I was looking to upgrade my Honda CB200.

It was quite disturbing to watch our precious motorbikes hauled into the air wrapped in chains on the Isle of Man Steam Packet Company Ferry. They clanged together as they were moved. If that wasn't traumatic enough, riding off the ferry was even worse, around and around a slippery helter-skelter of a ramp, wet with rain and oil, the rear ends skidding out from under us and trying to miss the sliding bike in front. But the weather had brightened up, the hotel was clean and the lady who owned it treated us like family. I had a room to myself in the attic, cosy and with an awesome view over the Irish Sea.

I even had to buy Stan a postcard and make him write on it to send to his girlfriend. Mick didn't have anyone and neither did I.

The Isle of Man TT covers ten days of racing, the qualifying races take up the first week. The races are a time trial of around sixty-kilometre laps on public roads known as the Snaefell Mountain Course; the elevation rises around four hundred metres from sea level. The bikes are production bikes, so it is a great opportunity to see the bike of your dreams in action. I was there to watch the Honda CB400F. Once the road is closed you can't move. We had a reasonably good spot watching from a pub car park. Bends on Snaefell where the most spectacular crashes would be most likely to occur were already crowded out early on race days. The real reason for going to the Isle of Man is not so much to watch the races – but for Mad Sunday. Which falls on the Sunday between the qualifying races and before the final week of racing. On Mad Sunday anyone can race around the track. We all did.

Unfortunately I dropped my bike – not crashed, please note. I was standing and it fell out from under me. I didn't have the strength to hold it and certainly not the strength to pick it up once it was on the ground. Not much damage – the crash bar took most of the weight of the bike and bent. The real damage was the badly bent gear-change pedal. Stan rolled his eyes and asked what I thought I was going to do about it because I couldn't ride it like that and he knew I was broke.

I got him to help me get it up a hill to a bike shop and told him to skedaddle. Something I had to do on my own. I went into the shop, explained what had happened, plus the money problem, and maybe a small tear gathered in the corner of my eye. They fell over each other to fix the bike for me. The bloke at the counter made me tea and fed me chocolate biscuits.

There are some things girls can do that guys can't.

John Kidson won the formula three with the CB400F. Formula three is for two stroke engines up to 250 cc and four strokes up to 400 cc. The two strokes are considered faster machines with better acceleration but I had ridden Stan's Suzuki – and a two stroke was never going to be on my wish list. The formula one event was stopped after four laps because of the weather. For each race about half the bikes don't even finish, it is considered the most dangerous race in the world.

There *was* a moment… Stan and I almost got together but we both backed off; he had a girlfriend, and I was celibate, single and staying that way.

He did lend me his sleeping bag – I was going directly from the Isle of Man to Stonehenge for the free festival. Hawkwind were top of the bill that year. I had neither tent nor sleeping bag, but I *would* find someone I knew.

After leaving Douglas on the ferry where the bikes are loaded by flying, we rode together as far as Wolverhampton. Then I'm on my own heading southwest on the M5, easily five hours of riding and alone for the first time in ages.

The police were at the entrance to the field where the festival camp was set up. They tried turning me back, telling me it is illegal to ride off a road onto a field and vice versa. Some law about driving over grass. I got off and pushed it onto the field. They assure me I will get a fine every time I do it. The fines will be in the post.

I found some people I knew and crashed in their tent, it beat sleeping around a campfire. The mood was joyful, the weather less so, mud everywhere and a bit of tension as the Hell's Angels were supposed to be turning up. No wonder there was such a police presence. The Hari Krishnas were offering free food. They were there for the concert as well, and the solstice celebrations, but their chapatis are the best I ever tasted. The lentil stew less so; it needed some white powder of the least scorable kind – salt.

We heard the roar of the Angels' bikes before they arrived. I'm pretty sure Hell's Angels don't care about grass laws. In fact the police parted as they made their way through the camp and they headed for the lesbian quarter. No one was sure what was going on – if they camped there on purpose or just didn't know. There was no trouble from anyone other than police harassment all week.

I couldn't manage the camp toilets – well, I did for a pee, but for bigger jobs I took my bike to the layby conveniences just down the road and risked a fine each time. I couldn't push the bike over the mud so I rode it, but you know what? I didn't care. There were even American tourists taking photos. They didn't ask. I was washing my hair under a standpipe while they snapped away: "Geez, look at the hippie washing."

Word got back to me that Stan had decided to make his way to the festival after all. I waited all night by the entrance – he didn't come.

I had promised Mum I would be back early to accompany her to a dinner as Dad was laid up with his back, but I found a phone box and made my excuses. Roy would have to substitute – I was waiting for Stan. He never did arrive, and I rode home alone.

By the time I arrived, I was stuffed and collapsed into bed and stayed there. I heard something going on in the night but I rolled over and went back to sleep.

It was Stan. He had turned up looking for me. Mum had opened the door in her dressing gown, invited him in and made him bacon sandwiches. This is what she told me the next day; she never made me bacon sandwiches!

"What a nice boy," she said.

That afternoon he came back and apologised about Stonehenge. His Dad had told him the police were turning people away from the illegal festival. It wasn't illegal but the police tried to make it so, fearing damage and drug taking. The monument of Stonehenge was fenced off, and yes there were drugs – none taken by me I might add – but there wasn't any trouble. Everyone ignored the police and their weirdo driving-on-grass rules. The reason he had come to the house, he said, was to ask me out.

Our first date was to the movies. We saw different films. Dad asked what kind of courtship this was, and we said in unison, "A very sensible one given the price of cinema tickets." That's how it has been ever since.

Christmas comes and goes, I pass my Open University exams and sign up for the science foundation course S101, chemistry, biology, physics, and earth science. Apart from a biology 'O' level I have no idea at all about physics and earth science and have proved beyond doubt that I suck at chemistry.

Although I'm not on bed rest, I am keeping a low profile. Too scared to do anything, I can't feel the baby move and I spend half my time at the clinic or the GP getting the heartbeat picked up by the stethoscope. We have bought a second-hand TV. I really couldn't cope without one. Today, I wish we had never bothered because I'm home alone when I watch the final double-length episode of *M.A.S.H.* As it finishes and the theme track "Suicide is Dangerous" plays, I walk into the street, hugely pregnant, and traumatised, but no one is there. I can't even see any lights on to go and hit someone up for a cuppa. How could 20th Century Fox allow tragedy to befall so many members of the 4077th at the end of the war in Korea? *M.A.S.H.* used to be a comedy!

Chapter 18: This Could Have Been Avoided

I am sitting on the back doorstep in the sun working out the density of various rocks with a bucket of water, a stick and a cup. Last night I had a ten pence coin fixed to a stick with a bit of plasticine working out the diameter of the moon. S101 only started five weeks ago. They sent me a huge, sturdy cardboard box packed with polystyrene drawers. It houses all manner of chemicals and bits of kit for the home experiments. The old lady I met in Loughborough said if I wanted something badly enough then I could do it. Everything is going well but the niggling pain is turning into outright agony as I rock to and fro on the doorstep, attempting to get the first assignment completed before I give up and agree that I'm in labour.

Naturally it stops as soon as I get to Gravesend Hospital. Given the car crash, the bed rest and all the other drama, they are not keen to send me home. The due date is still a week away, but they tell me I will need a caesarean due to pelvic insufficiency. I have been to the most recent antenatal classes, and I know the number of caesareans carried out in this hospital are more than the average so I am not giving in without a fight. I insist that I'm allowed what they call a trial labour. They clearly think I am a nuisance. We agree I will be induced first thing in the morning. This is a large and busy ward. There isn't any chance of sleep here and Stan is sent home and told there is no need to come back until at least tomorrow afternoon.

Gosh, the night is long, with screaming, torches shining in my eyes to see if I'm asleep, gas tanks clanging together as they get changed and yes… even snoring! How can anyone sleep through this? I am completely exhausted – and worse still, I don't get breakfast. They are convinced I will soon be begging for a caesarean. My chin is set in the determined mode I am known for. I have got this!

While everyone else is having breakfast, a nurse inserts a prostaglandin pessary into my vagina; it will dissolve and soften the cervix. Almost immediately I have diarrhoea. I leave a trail of poo through the ward as I run to the loo and the pessary drops into the toilet. Since that wasn't the desired outcome, I am set up with a drip. I want to get the results of my experiment written up. I can't be late with my first assignment.

Nothing is happening in terms of either the labour or the assignment. I'm hungry, and my focus is poor. My failed maths O-level is no help to me either. Our maths teacher was female, the daughter of a miner, and you would have thought she would have some empathy with us scholarship girls. If you didn't know what you were doing, then you weren't welcome in her class. I certainly didn't know what I was doing. I had asked to do extra English, maths and French, but I wasn't deemed stupid enough.

Lunchtime doesn't bring lunch, but I'm still not in the mood to quit. At least Stan turns up. He tries to help with my assignment but in the end, I send him to the shop to get the Daily Telegraph; I shall have a go at the quick crossword. My ultimate goal is the cryptic, way beyond my current skills.

At least I am in labour for certain, and coping. Putting my best face on, I can be quite persistent. They have moved me to a small room of my own – but the crossword is going badly and time is dragging. Nurses pop in to see how I am going and report a distinct lack of progress. I don't know what that means; something must be happening, considering all this gut wrenching.

We grind on towards dinnertime… which I also don't get. A nurse has come up with some glycerine mouth swabs, which help enormously since I haven't even been allowed a drink. I am hampered by tea withdrawal. I drink a lot of tea. I used to drink coffee, but pregnancy put paid to that.

I haven't eaten for 24 hours. Luckily I am not one to get grumpy. Stan gets tetchy if he even misses morning tea; he wouldn't cope with this at all. Then an almighty wail goes up next-door and there is crying and howling, the like of which I never heard before. A nurse bursts through the door to let me know the lady in the next room has delivered a dead baby. Her husband knew the baby had died. She hadn't been told because they thought she might lose the will to push, requiring a caesarean. Not in her best interest. Ironic, then, that they are trying to push me into agreeing to one.

The compromise on my part is a wire up my vagina screwed to my baby's head to monitor the heartbeat. I prefer the ultrasound, or even an ear trumpet but I can tell they want to get the most out of the machines that go beep. Intervention wasn't in my plan, and to be honest I feel beaten. I can't do the crossword, my assignment isn't complete, I haven't been fed or even had a cup of tea, and I am not making progress. I can sense two things from the staff; they are losing patience with me (some didn't have any to start with), and I detect a sense of urgency with one dead infant on this shift already.

I agree to pethidine. I am assured that reducing the pain will speed things up and they tell me my baby is getting stressed. Not part of my plan either.

This is the worst decision ever because within two minutes I have lost all sense. I can see unrecognisable faces grotesquely looming in and out, and their words have no meaning. I cannot understand what they want from me, and I begin to panic. Then they panic as the monitor stops beeping, and they grab the bed and drag it out the door. Stan is left alone. Someone shouts to him, but I don't understand what they say. These ugly-faced bodies are running the bed along the corridor, we enter an incredibly brightly lit room, and I hear the first words that make sense and yet they don't make any sense.

"It's too late."

"Too late for what?" I scream.

"It's all right, love, the baby has moved too far for a caesarean. We are doing a forceps delivery. Keep calm, baby will be out in a minute."

Stan misses the delivery, abandoned when they ran with the bed. I am out of my mind, but the sudden delivery and the colossal amount of blood and general debris has sharpened my focus. I don't even see the baby; a nurse tells me baby has gone to SCBU. Because of the car crash I already understand this means special care baby unit.

There is a whole load of cleaning up going on. The lights are so bright and I realise I'm in a theatre. My plan, formed through antenatal classes and extra reading, was nothing like this. I ask that the lights be turned off or at least down, and they do it. The nurses are giving me a bit of a bed bath but tell me not to get too comfortable because my night is far from over.

"There is a lot of damage down below, love. It'll take a bit of stitching. Rest up, lovey."

"Stan?" It's a bit of a quiver slash plea. I want him badly.

"No, love. We sent him home – he needs his rest too."

"Does he? Does he really?" I am too overcome to fight about it.

The stitching doctor is from Saudi Arabia. He is calm, softly spoken, and happy to work in the half-light. It really is late now. The baby… I have to say baby because I'm still confused. I thought someone said it was a boy, which can't be right because I am expecting a girl. Until I'm sure, this baby who can't be named was born at 9ish. If I heard right and it is a boy, then Stan and I are still arguing over Matthew or Zach. I am in the Zach camp.

While he is stitching, we chat. There has been a big focus on female circumcision in the UK recently and a push to ban the practice. There are a variety of operations – a loose term to describe mutilation of the genitalia of young girls. Different countries have different practices; some, such as Somalia, use the skin from the labia to seal the vagina over in almost all their girl children between the ages five to eleven. You can imagine the problems with peeing and everything else. The covering then needs to be cut for sex or childbirth and is often resealed, so the mutilation doesn't stop once it has begun. A prospective husband will examine his child bride to ensure she is sealed and no one else has been there. Even the female relatives get involved in examining the girl's bits to ensure everything is still secure down there.

In other countries they leave the vagina open but cut out any sensitive tissue, essentially the bits you can see (or enjoy). As my stitching goes past the hour, I'm concerned with what I will have left. He explains the emergency forceps left what he describes as a disaster scene. He is doing his best to make a good job. He tells me his sister had to be circumcised to find a good husband; a Saudi man won't be interested in an intact woman. Because she can't work, her only hope is to marry well. He has two daughters of his own and he tells me it is a terrible conflict. The girls are growing up in the UK. Mutilations are carried out here, but I suspect most blokes in the UK won't be looking for that sort of thing. He still feels the pull of the culture, the horror and shame it will bring on the family if he doesn't do it. Yet he knows there is only pain and misery to come from it for his girls.

I'm practically asleep as he ties the last knot and delivers the final blow. "All of this could have been avoided, you know?"

I stare at him through the gloom. I feel guilty enough about today's effort and now I sense an impending lecture about the caesarean that was ordered yesterday (actually, since it is gone midnight technically it was the day before yesterday).

"Your baby is fine. His heart never stopped and there was never an emergency the monitor lead broke."

I can't process what he is saying but I have latched on to the fact that *his* heart was the term used. "His back?" I ask and the doctor looks puzzled.

"His back is fine. He has two arms, two legs and all the fingers and toes. You don't want to see him now – he is a bit beaten up. You need some sleep and so do I. Make the most of a night off."

I don't really want a night off – I thought an immediate breastfeed was important – but my head is still in a serious mess from the pethidine, and I feel it could get into the breast milk. The fact he would already have got it via my placenta hasn't crossed my mind.

I finally get taken to the ward and I do get a bit of sleep. They bring my severely swaddled baby to the bedside in a plastic box on wheels. Immediately I have a sneaking suspicion that someone has pulled a crafty swap. Firstly, everyone said I was expecting a girl. This boy baby has dark-yellow skin, with significant bruising and a hole in his square forehead. At least I get breakfast which takes my mind off the poor boy.

A photographer turns up; apparently everyone wants a photo of their baby. We both look at the infant sleeping peacefully (drugged) in the plastic box. She can't hide the expression on her face.

"Don't worry, lovey, we can do something with him." She busies herself in her bag of tricks and masks the bruising with some makeup. His head is still square, yellow and has a hole in it. She can't disguise everything. She takes a few shots and is off to mothers with better looking babies.

A nurse appears. "Baby will need changing," she sings and disappears. Stan had practised on Julie's kid next door; I haven't a clue. Unwrapping him like a giant sweet, I find he has a little blue wrist band, quite tight around his chubby, dark-skinned arm. Stan and I are both very fair. The card at the end of the plastic box states, "Male infant 8lb 9oz forceps full term". Definitely male as I explore under the nappy.

Since I woke him up with the unwrapping he has been quite wriggly, so his back isn't broken. As I lie him down he pees a strong arc of urine directly into his open mouth. I am horrified and realise how totally unprepared I am for all of this.

Then Stan bowls in. He doesn't care about visiting hours after last night's drama and he has no trouble folding a nappy and shows me how they work best for boy babies. Luckily Julie had a boy.

"A bit of piss in the gob never hurt anyone," he says. "Oh yes, there is a letter for you." He hands me a thick envelope. My state finals are next Wednesday.

They won't let me out. I think it's because everyone in the hospital wants to look at my stitched bits. It seems like a parade.

"Do you mind?" they ask.

Of course I bloody mind, but this is a teaching hospital. Until they tell me one of the psych students wants to see… then I draw the line. Cheekier still, it is sleazy Terry! What the hell! There is no earthly reason he should look at my twat and I won't even see him.

I tell the nurse that he can, "Fuck off." I don't usually get so annoyed. Stan has soothed things by bringing in toilet paper. Newspaper would be an improvement on the shiny stuff provided here. The other women on the ward take the piss out of me but I don't smoke, I barely drink – I am entitled to soft toilet paper.

The women in this six-bed ward are disgusting. Three of them spit grape pips about the place and say the cleaners are paid to clean. They had some sparkling wine last night and popped corks around the babies in the plastic cribs.

There is one I feel a bit sorry for. She is in the corner on the opposite side of the room, so I practically stare at her for most of the day, having nowhere else to gaze. Her husband came in to tell her he was leaving her. Which is bad enough, but now her five-year-old daughter has been admitted to intensive care in a bad way, according to the paediatrician that came to see her. The pathetic curtain allows no privacy. As soon as she told him she didn't understand how the girl could get sick because she sterilises everything she has. I heard a huge sigh from him. The girl has just started school; I imagine she has zero resilience to anything and will pick up everything in a classroom full of virus-laden new-entrants.

I want out – but they think I should stay for a week. I can't risk it; I need to be at the nursing school in time for the exam. I feel dreadful – I'm weak and exhausted, and my stitches hurt like hell – but I put some blusher on my cheeks and push for my release.

151

They relent. Stan can come and get me on Monday, so I will have been here five days since the birth, a week since admission. Sunday is Mothers' Day; everyone has visitors and flowers. No one comes to see me, including Stan, so no flowers. I think my hormones are a mess because all I do all day is cry. The woman in the corner bed cries all day as well.

We have put the house up for sale. I have to drive past the crash site every day and I can't shake it from my mind.

Chapter 19: Marking Time

Exam day is interesting. I have a pillow with me, in deference to the stitches. Revision has been haphazard because I hadn't thought I would make the March sitting. Neither did I expect to find Joan there. She failed in November. Sad, but her reaction on seeing me is bizarre, making a huge fuss. The exam can't start on time because she is insisting that I can't be here due to being on maternity leave. The invigilator ends up phoning the nursing council who confirm I have every right to be here, and that we should continue. I have no idea why she would even care.

I leave as soon as the exam is over, I know I have done enough to pass and that is all that matters. I don't want to discuss it with her, I have a week-old baby and I need to get into some kind of routine. I have five weeks' leave left, I must sort out a baby minder and we need to prepare to move.

Time flies by. Stan can't have any leave to help but he does help, hugely. Even so, I'm alone a lot and convinced I'm doing things wrong. Breastfeeding is difficult and then there are the stitches. I walk for hours with Zach in the pram. I don't know what else to do.

Joan failed again and blames me for upsetting her concentration!

With my six weeks of maternity leave over, I have returned to Joyce Green to fix up the lost hours following the car crash. I'm happy with the directive that my time is spent here, given my interest in maternal mental health. It is further to travel than the other admission units but there aren't any nightshifts, making the baby care arrangements easier. Zach is not a happy baby, I am not an earthmother, and this weekend we have moved even further away. The only plus is that if we'd stayed there, each day I would have been travelling the only road out of the area, passing my power pole – which we ended up having to pay for and we didn't even get the old one. After all

153

the work we did getting the nursery ready, Zach never saw it. Sleep deprived and living out of boxes, I feel everything is conspiring against me.

The new house is much older than our first cookie-cutter home. We will have to put heating in – either a gas boiler or coal fire – but we are OK about installing radiators and all that. Dad did it when we were kids, and I paid attention. The house has three big bedrooms, two lounges and a massive garden. The downside is the only toilet is off the kitchen. I'm not sure we can do anything about that. If we stay we will have to take a bit out of a bedroom to make an upstairs bathroom.

It is also on a slip road off the main drag to the power station. Better for Stan – but it is a busy road. Plus, the garden path is overgrown with conifers down one side. I am allergic to them, so they must go. There's a lot to do, but the garage is big enough to drive the car in and still be able to open the door to get out. That will be a novelty.

—∧∧—

Ward Sister remembers me from my previous placement and volunteered to take me for the extra hours, happy to have some qualified hands. This is a bit previous because although I passed the exam, I can't register until the extra time is made up. Sister is not paying any heed to this small issue.

I have been here a week; the days are a blur since the nights are as well. Today I gave one of our patients her regular depot injection. This is an oil based antipsychotic preparation; it disperses over four weeks for this lady. Injections are more convenient especially where patients are likely to forget to take pills or decide not to. It is hard to suck an injection out. She had been on leave for the long May Day weekend. She seemed cheerful and practically ready for discharge. Now she's dead, and this might bite both Sister and me on the bum! I am qualified to give injections without supervision, but it is at least seven months since I've done so. Being rusty meant triple checking everything – right drug, right dose, right patient, right time, method all good. It went like clockwork and ordinarily the lady in question is a bit ratty. We have met a few times over the last three years, but today she was cheerful, grateful even. This was my last job before the shift change, she died before I finished the paperwork. I am rostered off for three days now. Leaving everyone else to deal with the body, I grab my jacket and go. She will surely have to go to the coroner. Thank goodness my bike has a battery the size of a car battery and it will start. I couldn't be using a kick start or worse running down the road and leaping on it like I had to with the old one.

At home I'm a cot case, having killed someone, yet needing to be a mother. It is extremely tough – we don't have any family near enough to help. The phone doesn't ring even though I sit next to it when I am not out. I put Zach in the pram and walk. I am walking miles. The three days pass slowly.

On day four I drop Zach at the babyminder, and drive straight to the hospital in the mini, with no heart or strength for my Guzzi. The news is surprising though. No one is blaming me. The patient had taken a large overdose of codeine, presented herself to A&E and told them. They dismissed her because she has turned up a dozen times before and it has never been true. She is a documented time waster. They didn't even alert the MHU, which you would think they might have done given she was an inpatient on leave. My injection made no difference to her outcome.

I am too exhausted to take it all in, so I cry.

Sister is kind but firm. We have another admission – a simple job. This lady was a regular to the ward years ago but now her daughter looks after her at home. The thing is the daughter needs a hysterectomy so is booking Mum in for a couple of weeks' holiday. As a carer she is entitled to help in the form of respite care for her mother for exactly this sort of thing. Ordinarily her mother would go to one of the old folks' homes, but because she has been diagnosed with schizophrenia they are not keen to take her. I get a bit fed up with inappropriate placements, but I guess if she knows the

155

place already she will be comfortable with young and very unwell people.

She is quite a large lady with white hair, a smiley face and twinkly cornflower-blue eyes. Her daughter tells me she has had zero sign of schizophrenia for many years; she is simply old and forgetful and can't be left home alone so here she is. Luckily we have an empty single room – quite a rarity – so she can at least have some quiet space. Despite her size she is mobile and doesn't need care with showering or anything of that nature – just a bit of company, regular meals and a bed.

I complete the paperwork and check her out physically, pulse and blood pressure. It's been a while since I have done an admission, so I should have made myself a checklist. I think I have done everything. The students look to me because they think I'm qualified yet I've been out of the loop for long enough to have forgotten most of what I learned, plus I am sleep deprived and have baby brain. Which way is up, is anyone's guess.

I go home and walk. The Mother and Baby Unit is empty. I might be the next guest.

—∿—

Because the birth was such a disaster I have a lot of stitches – a hundred and twenty-eight, to be exact. There isn't a league table, but I know it is a big number. So on Tuesdays my GP has a fiddle about, cauterising things, or at least that's what he says. He has told me I need to try it out, see if things down below are in working order. The Saudi Arabian guy that did the stitching was sweet but his words still ring in my head.

"All of this could have been avoided, you know? Your baby is fine, his heart never stopped, there was never an emergency, the monitor lead broke."

So, Tuesday afternoons are the sequelae of a cock-up. My GP has told me to try it out and so I will. Not sure what shift Stan is on; he needs to participate!

There is a block course later in the year at Reading University, but we need a lab day earlier, so off I trot to the local high school, leaving Stan in charge. I have never met the others, but we are assigned to groups and our experiments are going well. No one is seriously annoying and when we see the instructions for the next experiment requiring us to leave vanadium boiling for an hour, naturally we decide to go to the pub for lunch.

When we get back, we have a surprise test. And it *was* a surprise because one of the questions was to describe the colour changes the vanadium went through as it boiled. Another cock-up. Though I am only partially responsible for this one.

—∿—

The respite-care old lady is enjoying the attention she is getting from the youngsters. Her daughter has had her operation, and everything is fine. But today the old lady slipped over. I don't know what made her fall. It takes six of us to get her up. Her ankle is swelling already, this doesn't look good. We try an ice pack, a cup of tea, the usual stuff, but in the end Sister has the Registered Nurse take her to X-ray in a wheelchair. The ankle is broken. The old lady doesn't want to stay in her room – she thinks no one will visit. She is being spoilt in the lounge where she can interact with the others. She seems happy, but it takes a bit of explaining to her daughter who is not best pleased and unable to visit – she is still recovering on the ward from her surgery.

We needn't have worried; the youngsters are keeping her entertained. I must give another routine injection. I'm trying to keep my nerves under wraps. Everyone keeps telling me about getting back on the horse, but the last person is dead, regardless of why, and I feel the weight of responsibility. This woman is so thin, and an intramuscular injection requires I find some muscle. Sister agrees the usual upper outer quadrant of her bum, is not meaty enough. "Try her thigh," she says. So, I do, and the needle hits the bone and bends. At least I manage to get it out and I am praised for my quick thinking, but I still feel like a failure.

—∿—

Broken ankle lady is complaining of stomach-ache. It is difficult to get her up. I'm sure if I sat about all day I wouldn't feel so good. Between us we make sure she does move but the pains are getting worse. She is having a hard time trying to convey how she feels. We have assumed all along there is nothing wrong with her mental state, now we don't know.

Sister calls in a doctor who is not happy about her bowel sounds, or lack thereof. He asks for the bowel book. What? Oh yes, on Female Hospital we did keep a bowel book – we wrote down who went and when – but on this ward everyone is fit and attends to their own needs. If this lady had gone to an old folk's home for her respite, then perhaps they would have kept a book. None of us can remember the last time her bowels would have been working and she can't remember either.

So, he organises a trip to X-ray – twice now in a week for the same patient who shouldn't even be here. She died while she was there. Bowel blockage. We had been entrusted with her respite and we killed her. Not one of us, all of us. Technically I will soon be registered. I passed all my practical assessments; I passed the state exam and there are just over two weeks until I have made up the time. The award ceremony is later in the year. Am I capable of being a Registered Nurse and all it entails? Not at all. My confidence has taken a dive, and I don't think I should have responsibility for my baby, let alone a ward full of sick people.

Then things get worse. I can't stop throwing up.

It is 6 a.m., and there is a frantic rapping. The baby has only just gone to sleep – have a heart. The noise is difficult to ignore. So early – it can't be for a good reason.

A glimpse at my reflection in the hallway mirror highlights a nightdress streaked with breastmilk and baby puke. The thin summer dressing gown should have been washed; I'd been banking that no one would see it. I look like I haven't slept in a year, and, overwhelmed by nausea, I could be pregnant.

Stan is on nightshift at the power station. The banging is at the front door that no one uses. My heart sinks; smart blue police uniforms are wrapped around two giant-sized guys.

Anticipating tragic news, I'm caught off guard when one of them says, "Where is your gate?"

I hear their words, but my first-time-mother brain fog causes me to pause. These gentlemen are concerned about my gate?

Their heads turn, pointedly, towards the driveway, eyebrows rising. One gate is missing, but my mind is beginning to rally. "That's right. I broke in, during the night, using the gate as a ladder."

"May I ask why?"

"I went to investigate a noise, and the kitchen door slammed behind me. Without keys I couldn't get back in, and the baby was locked inside."

I lead the cops around the back to show them – and it isn't there! Some bastard has stolen our gate. Fortunate, then, that the police are here.

Leaving easy access for would-be-robbers wasn't clever, but it was too heavy to lug back, especially in the dark. I'd already damaged the thing dragging it that far. The gates are distinctive, steel made to look like wrought iron. I loathe them, but they do the job. Side on, a gate makes a remarkably stable ladder.

But the police already know it has gone *and* where it is. They demand to know what I have been doing since 5 a.m. I take the cops back into the house by the back door and describe my early morning feeding and burping routine but I can see it isn't impressing them.

"So, what did you hear, since you admit you were awake?"

"Like what?" I'm searching for clues.

"Like someone driving a tractor through the wall of the post office. Then coming around to the back of your house, stealing the gate, tying a safe to it, attaching it to a tractor and dragging it down the road. It would have caused sparks, and it has damaged the road surface. Those old safes are lined with stone for fireproofing. They weigh a ton!" He stares directly into my face. "Your gate is in the ditch at the bottom of the hill."

"Tractor?"

"Yes. We can tell from the tyre marks."

How can I have failed to hear it? Even asleep, the sound should have penetrated my brain. They can't seriously suspect me – I'm unable to keep track of my keys, let alone arrange a safe-stealing event. Plus, I don't have a tractor.

The post office is less than a hundred metres away. It all would have made a fair amount of noise – hardly a ram-raid, but similar.

Although not at peak performance, I am smarter than to use my own gate in a getaway. Was the gate stolen because they intended to use it anyway, i.e. the theft was premeditated, or did they get the safe as far as our house and think "*Some kind of sled would make dragging this thing easier,*" meaning the theft was opportunistic?

My mind immediately flashes to the lyrics of "Alice's Restaurant". The protagonists in this Arlo Guthrie anti-US-draft song are put in a cell by Officer Obie and charged with littering, as evidenced by a load of photographs. Obie takes their belts in case they hang themselves. I don't have a belt; maybe the cops will take my shoelaces.

It seems odd for a master criminal to wander around a random garden in the hope of finding something to use following a ram-raid. Why not take the gate in the driveway? Did they know where the other gate was?

The policemen show me eight-by-ten colour glossy photographs with circles and arrows and a paragraph on the back of each one explaining what each one was, to be used as evidence – "sled gate in ditch, Power Station Road" and "matching gate in situ at 17 Vague Villas". One of them takes my fingerprints, then says, "Wait… "

My sleepy brain is back with Officer Obie in Stockbridge, Massachusetts. My alibi is paper thin.

They don't want my shoelaces. They say my fingerprints are the only ones on the gate. I believe them even though it can't be true. They will find whatever supports their narrative.

At that moment Stan arrives, and we go through the whole story.

"Bugger the gate," says Stan. "What about the robbery a few weeks ago – the grinder and jigsaw? You have an eyewitness, and you haven't done a thing."

"With respect, sir, major crime must take precedence over petty theft. Your power tools are listed. If they turn up in our enquiries you will see them again."

I am upset – not so much for the grinder, but my jigsaw was brand new, and I'd had to watch the creeps from down the road steal it. The first power tool of my own. I have been teaching myself to make wooden toys, starting with a petrol station including a ramp to a roof carpark. Using sleek modern drawer handles as barriers so the cars wouldn't fall off was a touch of genius. I imagined starting a toy business. My attempt to save juggling a baby and a full-time job.

I hadn't been up to confronting burglars, even though I knew who they were. With the phone downstairs, and being alone with a baby in the house, I was too scared to move. My police report lists the address of the thieves!

We are down a gate, held by the police as evidence – which we may eventually get back – a jigsaw I'm emotionally attached to, and a grinder on its last legs. I doubt we will see those again. It hadn't been worth the excess on the insurance to make a claim.

Plus, it is Tuesday. GP day.

Figure 6. The Friern Hospital

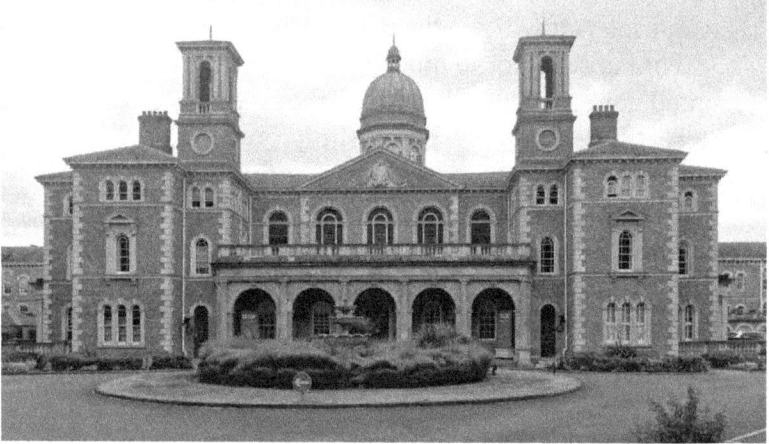

Chapter 20: Sinking

Stan is taking care of Zach, giving me the opportunity to walk to the surgery in the sun. Most people would drive. The pavement is uneven, and in some places absent where it gives way to earth. Often it is slushy mud but now baked dry in the summer sun. It takes around thirty minutes, and to me it feels like a treat. I'm OK, but not thrilled at the prospect of more poking about down below. I push open the surgery doors, a few minutes late and a little puffed, but I can go straight in.

My GP seems satisfied with his explorations.

I tell him I feel nauseous.

"Have you given things a go, as I suggested?" he asked.

"Once. Weeks ago, when you suggested it."

"But you are still breastfeeding?"

"Trying to," I tell him. "I'm finding it hard, what with working, moving house, and now our gate is involved in that post office job."

He raises an eyebrow. "I doubt you could be pregnant then. You're probably just run down."

He isn't wrong there, plus I have been walking many miles a day on top of work. I don't know what else to do. Zach appears to enjoy it; he is settling down. The baby-minder had got to the point where she was going to say she couldn't have him.

"You should try and relax, get more rest – sleep when Zach sleeps. Make an appointment for next Tuesday. Things really are improving, you know."

But I don't know.

I put my knickers back on and leave the room. The receptionist is busy writing when I say I need another appointment.

She doesn't look up. "Name please."

The silence forces her to look up. "I need your name." As if by way of explanation.

I cannot think – overtaken by the inquisition.

163

"Address then, lovey?" Her face has softened as she realises my struggle.

At that moment the community midwife walks past. "Are you OK?" She puts an arm around my shoulder.

It is enough to make me cry. "I have no idea," I tell her.

She turns to the receptionist. "I was expecting this," she says. "Get hold of her husband." She writes down his name and guides me into her office.

I explain how Zach was swapped at birth. I tell her about the dead baby in the next room and how I never saw my baby. Then the next day they tried to tell me the yellow, square-headed child was mine. I told her about the dead patients, the move, the police, everything.

By the time I stop sobbing Stan and Zach have arrived. Zach's wearing a familiar expression.

The midwife looks at me. "He has your face and your pout."

I can't argue with her. Not one of my best looks either.

She turns to Stan. "She is going to have to have time off work and so are you. This isn't uncommon. She didn't react well to pethidine, and the birth experience wasn't what we wanted either. Take her home and put her to bed."

I don't mind the sound of that.

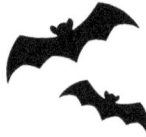

I sleep like a log, relieved that someone knows I am not finding motherhood the happy ever after I dreamt of for so long. I'm feeling guilty though, I should be grateful – and I am. Zach is perfect – his head is no longer square and yellow – but nothing is the way I thought it would be. Stan promised us a second breakfast, but we seem to be waiting. He is hesitant, in two minds I would say.

Then two "suits" walk through the door. One is my GP. The other I don't know.

The stranger talks directly to Stan. "We will take her to the unit, but you need to sign the papers."

"Papers?" says Stan.

164

"The Mental Health Act – it requires two doctors. I'm Doctor Sweeny, a psychiatrist, and we have Doctor Bowden, her General Practitioner, and under the terms of the Act we need one relative. That's you."

"No, that's not me," says Stan. "You have this all wrong."

My GP intervenes. "Stan, you have to agree this has been coming for a while. It was a traumatic birth which sometimes precipitates psychosis. We need to work together – she didn't know who she was the other day at the surgery."

"I'm not doing it. I will not get involved with locking her up." Stan is adamant.

I don't exist, obviously, since they are talking as if I am not here.

The psychiatrist has more to say. "Let's get her mother involved – mothers always sign."

I think Stan is going to explode. Mr. Cool – the one who sorted everything when we were teenagers, who could be relied upon to get us a ride home, get the ambulance if needed. Whatever wanted sorting, he would sort it, and here is a stranger thinking they can muscle in.

"What she needs is sleep!"

Ever the conciliator, my GP suggests medication. Delving into his bag, he gives Stan a bottle of pills. "Haloperidol," he says. "It will make a world of difference. I will pop back in a couple of days. If we don't treat her, she will stay crazy."

I give Stan *the look*.

"She's pregnant," he says. "She won't be taking those."

He is buying time. I'm smart enough to know I am better off saying nothing.

The psychiatrist rolls his eyes. "In that case we also need to sort out a termination or you will have two babies and a crazy wife. When was your last period?"

At last, he turns to face me, but my GP butts in. "Don't ask."

"Over my dead body, and you can all get out!" Stan thrusts the door open and shoos everyone away.

We watch them leave; I don't know if I am watching help walk away.

I need to get my shit in a heap.

"Second breakfast!" says Stan. "The café by the river. We could do with some fresh air."

I put on some cleanish clothes. Stan grabs the sleeping baby and pushchair, and we are out the door. The morning sun casts fresh light on a black start. When we get to the café, I order unfertilised eggs on toast. It's obvious, even to me, I can't cope.

—⋀—

The nursing school are furious. I must complete the time, and they can't put my name forward for graduation until I have. Graduation is not far away. When can they expect me to get my sorry arse back to work?

When I stop crying, walking, throwing up… I don't know is the honest answer.

I go back to my GP and agree to go into the Medway mental health mother and baby unit with Zach in three days' time.

Except I have a bad feeling, so I phone the unit the night before admission day. I need reassurance but it isn't forthcoming. The cot has gone, they have a bed for me they are quick to tell me –, it is essential I am treated – but I can't bring Zach. I must go or I risk hospitalisation against my will.

I know Stan won't be involved but they *will* find someone. I am not leaving Zach, even with Stan. Since he has my expression, and not one of my prettier ones, he must be mine and he needs me. Even if I'm not much cop.

Stan has another idea.

"Sweets, would a holiday help?"

"A holiday would always help but how can we? They want me back at work, we have a baby, it sounds too hard."

"Yes, but would it help?"

"Hhhmmm, ideas?"

"I read about sailing courses, they aren't as expensive as you might think, safety in the water and all that, it's a government push to stop Brits killing themselves at sea. What do you think?"

I don't have to think for long, I have always been interested in sailing.

Stan rings to book a weekend away at the Sailing Centre on the Isle of Wight, my parents can surely cope for a weekend? They tell him about a special deal. We can study for a dinghy sailing certificate, which is a whole week, for the same cost as the weekend course. The snag, they tell him, is it will be dormitory accommodation.

It sounds ideal.

The thought of getting away makes me feel happier, and I think I can face going back to work. The news on the ward is the announcement that the Friern will close, just as my training is ending. We have known since the 1960s. But the announcement has come as a total shock for the staff who work there – they found out on the evening news.

A glossy brochure Friern 2000 describing how the Friern would march into the future, a fanfare to modern mental health care, was produced only three years ago. Nothing has happened, but we feel it is the start of the long promise to empty the lunatics out of the asylums. I sense my three (extended) years may truly have been a waste. Colney Hatch (now the Friern) was based on the design of an Italian monastery and supposed to be a successor to the aging Bethlem Royal built in 1247. Treatment at Bethlem was degrading and brutal. For a small fee you could see the mad wretches chained and naked. This tourist destination closed in 1770, but things didn't improve. It has turned up in horror stories and films, most notably the Boris Karloff movie Bedlam in 1946. It was and is synonymous with madness. Bethlem Royal didn't close and is now held in high regard for its modern treatments. If that closes, then it really will be the end.

The sailing course is in six weeks; I will have made up the missing time by then. Everyone is concerned. I'm sent on a professional development course within the hospital grounds, meeting up with Sister for lunch. I think Sister put my name

167

forward so I wouldn't have to do shifts. She wants me to sleep at night; she knows I live a long way away and the evening shift means I don't get to bed until gone midnight.

Even then I don't think I sleep. Stan says the bed is his happy place. I watch him. His head hits the pillow and within minutes I can hear his soft, rhythmic breathing. I lie awake for what seems like hours, replaying the day on fast forward. When I eventually drift off I am flying, leaping from rooftop to rooftop and somersaulting up and down stairs. Sometimes I engage in wheelchair gymnastics where I have lost the use of my legs. Then come the videos, replaying the worst parts of my life in colour, complete with sound and smell. I wake exhausted. Stan is refreshed after doing nothing all night. How does that work?

Mum had me sedated when I was three months old. To be fair, it wasn't her suggestion. She didn't have any help. Few people had phones or cars and although in those days daughters often lived in the same street as their mother, this wasn't the case for us. Mum was on her own with a baby that didn't sleep and didn't stop screaming. I think the screaming had a lot to do with chilblains; I was born in the summer but still had to wear mittens all the time. Now I am older and suffer chilblains in my fingers and sleep with gloves throughout the year; I know how painful they can be. After three months Mum lost the plot. Advice at the time was to leave the baby in a pram at the end of the garden; our garden must have been too short. After being locked in a room for a weekend (the suggestion of the GP who assured her it would sort me out), I was diagnosed with brain too active for body and prescribed phenobarbitone (prescribed for epilepsy, which I don't have) until my body could catch up.

I have never heard such rubbish. When I asked Mum about it she said that as a new mother of a crying baby it was music to her ears to be told there was a medical issue that could be easily sorted with a chemical straitjacket. We emigrated to Australia when I was four and ran out of drugs enroute. The Australian doctor refused to give phenobarbitone to a child without epilepsy and told her to take me to kindergarten. We didn't last quite a year Mum simply found it too tough, but I never got sedated again.

I can't stop throwing up. All I can do is suck on slices of apple. I end up leaving Zach with Mum and Dad while we go to the Isle of Wight off the south coast. Dad is so proud, manhandling the pushchair; he would never have done that back in the day! Stan has passed his driving test, but we still have the heap-of-shit Mini which struggles to get us to Portsmouth where we leave it, we don't need it on the island and the cost of putting it on the ferry isn't worth it.

In my mind I hadn't linked being pregnant with having another baby. Not until the Sailing Centre. The week is an absolute hoot, the girls' dorm every bit as naughty as St Trinian's, even though we all count as adults. On the final night we go to a disco, ferried by a rubber rescue boat. It barely sits above the waterline, packed with all of us sailing students. When we leave late at night the tide has gone out and we drop several feet off the jetty in the dark, landing unceremoniously in the bottom of the boat. At *that* moment I equate being pregnant with having another baby. Without freaking out.

The next thing in my busy schedule is the block course for the lab work. I don't think they know I was in the group that stuffed up lab day. This time Stan drops me at Reading University, and I have organised a room close to the loo. I like science a lot more than I expected, and although I would not have knowingly put myself in this position when I enrolled, I manage. My grades aren't great, but a pass is a pass. I have the exam in December, and I know I'm better at exams than completing assignments. One of the things my posh school taught me was how to pass exams. Biology, Brain and Behaviour (SD286) can wait – I am not daft enough to enrol again next year. Two babies and possible mental deterioration following the birth will be enough, I'm not right in the head even now. Just a bit less worse, is how I might describe things.

I am noticeably pregnant when I eventually graduate. The Nursing Education woman makes no bones about her annoyance when I collect my certificate and badge. It took four years of effort to get one baby and one moment of seeing if everything was still in working order to get the second. Breastfeeding as a contraceptive is clearly overrated.

I am not in a fit state to work. The previous three and a half years replaced a serviceable brain with a rubbish one.

I'm not prepared to risk the previous performance. I have agreed to the aging (and condemned) All Saints Hospital. By the due time I am huge, and bored. The clinic tells me to make an appointment for the following week. When I try, they tell me the following Monday is Easter and the clinic will be closed. The clinic is only held on Mondays so I make an appointment for the next week after that. Surely I won't last? A baby couldn't be that overcooked?

The day before the appointment, and now three weeks overdue, I knock the coalbunker down with a sledgehammer. Nothing happens.

At the clinic they are cross. I don't feel I am to blame. I will be admitted in the morning and should expect a caesarean since the head is not engaged, the baby is big, and the old tale of pelvic insufficiency is once again rearing its ugly head.

I recall passing out in a shop doorway a few weeks ago after a bout of somersaulting – the baby, that is, not me; I don't do gymnastics in waking time. I knew the head couldn't be engaged.

They speak to me as if I am an infant, and it gets worse when I refuse both pain relief and monitoring. "If you want to listen, use an ear trumpet," I tell the nurse.

Stan is sent home. Nothing going on, they tell him. At least they don't go the pessary route; they give me an infusion and break my waters. I'm in pain, but I cannot make a fuss given the stance I have taken. They have no idea how stubborn I can be.

170

Stan and I are linked in ways we don't understand.

"This baby is coming, right now!" I announce. It's lunchtime and it isn't just because I'm not in favour of missing lunch, but truly, I can feel the head. A nurse puts me in a wheelchair and takes me to the lift. I am not a fan of the confined space and when it mysteriously descents to the basement I begin to panic. The nurse gets the elevator back to the ground floor birthing suite just as Stan shoots through the door in greasy overalls and Jade makes an exit with the cord wound around her neck twice. The midwife, still gripping her cheese sandwich, is wonderful and sorts the cord with a deft sleight of hand. Jade is the greenest and longest baby they have ever had, so naturally we call her String Bean. As the green fades it is replaced by yellow. She has a shock of black hair, and quite a tan under the green then yellow skin.

They won't let us go home and put us in the corridor under a dripping pipe because there is no room on the ward. At least I have her with me; no swapping this one out. They are waiting for me to crack, though they say they are observing her.

We spend a week doing nothing. Then I do crack. Not crazy – angry. She could have been out in the sun, which would improve her jaundice – the result of antibodies because of my rhesus-negative blood. Instead we lose a precious week in a corridor under a dripping pipe. Quite apart from the wet bed, it is like living on a motorway.

Jade is taken to the nursery every night or the plastic baby box will clog up the corridor. It is too busy at night as workers replace oxygen tanks and ferry equipment around. Plenty for me to watch while I'm not sleeping. They also bring her back regularly during the night for feeds. I have a feeling they are waking her up!

Bread tray transport

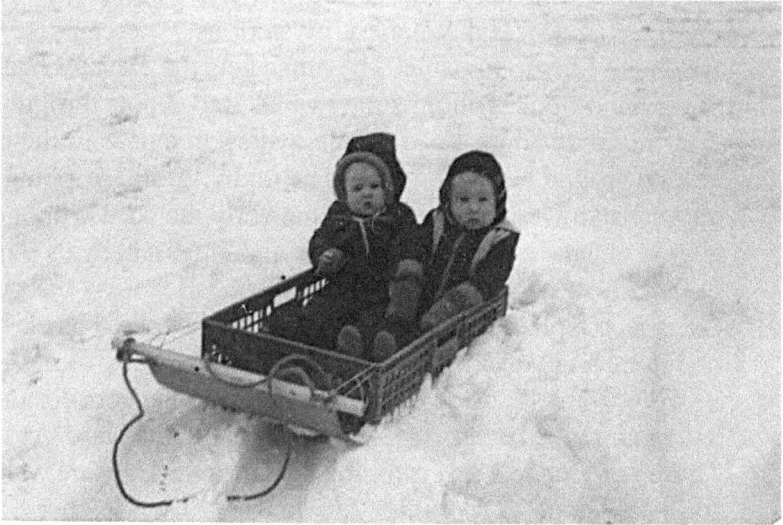

Personal photograph January 1985

Chapter 21: Going Solo

After the failure of breastfeeding as a contraceptive I have an IUD (intrauterine device) fitted. Stan hates it, says he can feel the string. The postnatal problems I was half expecting don't eventuate and I throw myself into being an apology for an earthmother. Swimming, tumble-time, even ice skating; toddlers and tiny chairs, terrifying. We skate to "Cecilia" played endlessly on a loop. It came out in 1970, but apparently it is brilliant ice-skating music. Zach wants it on at home all the time.

The IUD is a moot point anyway because Stan has scored himself a job in Saudi Arabia. It has been on the cards for a while. I could use my right of veto, but he isn't happy that he is coming up for a long-service award at the power station. He figures those are for old men and he isn't that person. For my part I have never felt settled in England, having felt the hot sands of Australia between my toes as a five-year-old. My friends say I was never meant to stay in England, and this employer is promising we will all be able to join Stan in Saudi in six months' time. There is no choice but to cope on my own for now.

I miss him dreadfully. He taped a load of stories for the kids before he left. Zach doesn't understand where he has gone but I'm not sure Jade even notices. There is a problem though – he gets paid a month in hand. Like most young couples with a mortgage, two babies and one income, we don't have a spare stash. We thought it would be hard enough to manage a month without income, but a month *in hand* means a two-month wait. Stan had to get a Saudi cheque drawn up on his payday. The day the cheque arrives in the post I'm down to zero in the bank account, and one egg, one tin of tuna fish and a handful of rice in the pantry.

The kids and I are waiting outside the bank for it to open. The children had half an egg each for breakfast; the rice and tuna fish were last night's dinner. I flourish the fancy-looking cheque at the bank manager and he says, "I can't accept that."

I almost pass out as he continues to explain, "Even if it looked less dodgy, it needs at least seven working days to clear."

I cry a lot more than I should, but I lack the energy and skills for much more. Between sobs I explain about the tin of tuna and the last egg. The bank manager forwards twenty pounds while the cheque clears and tells me that if it clears this time then they will make good immediately on further cheques and we won't have this problem.

Thank goodness the cheque does clear.

I am having a tough time though. Zach is on prophylactic antibiotics for chronic ear infection and Jade has become allergic to everything. Her clothes, the carpet, her car seat, and everything she eats and drinks results in spots. She also has asthmatic attacks usually winding up in hospital. Jade also doesn't sleep. Well, that's not true – she is asleep at seven each night but up at three a.m. That is the end of her night and nothing I do changes it. That's when her breathing's okay, of course. When it's not she's awake all the time (which I guess is a good thing). All her clothes are now cotton or silk. Her carpet and blinds have gone. I wash her bedding every day and wipe down her cot. I have sewn a cotton car seat cover and make everything she eats and drinks from scratch.

Now she has an ear infection too, but she has to have injections twice a day because she is allergic – not to the antibiotic itself, but to the syrup. I am not allowed to give her the injections, so I drag her through the snow in a green plastic bread-tray with hardboard nailed to the bottom. The pushchair won't work in the snow. With no one to mind Zach he is jammed into the bread tray next to her.

Zach doesn't speak. Jade is not yet a year old and does all the talking for him. She doesn't shut up. This was exactly how things played out with my brother except he is younger than me. It turned out he was deaf. I have taken Zach to the GP; he says there is nothing to be done about his ears until he is five.

Mum tells me to go back to the GP and bang on the desk and threaten to go private. So I do exactly that.

Threatening to go private works a treat! Miraculously we can be seen for free on the National Health Service right away, and the specialist deems his case urgent. Hospital speak for urgent is usually months, but he says within four weeks. I don't have much time to prepare Zach for it. His adenoids are removed and grommets are inserted into his ears, and while that happens I flip a table in the café because I am so stressed.

Walking back to the ward, after apologising and righting the table, I see Zach up ahead – standing on a mobile hospital bed and looking ready to duke it out with the porter who's pushing it. The specialist decides I should take him home. I need to note that he woke up before they had finished, and as it has happened once there is a chance it could occur in the future.

Before we leave, I get to talk to one of the other mums. Her son waited until he was five. He has been deaf all the while, and the fluid that built up in his sinuses over those years became compacted. During his operation, his sinuses were drained but collapsed and are now packed with gauze. The nurses will gradually remove the stuffing over the coming days. He will be in for at least a week. What a nightmare. Even Zach is going to need speech therapy at two years old. It would be a much bigger job at five, I would think.

There is a letter from Stan. "How do you fancy New Zealand?" He has been chatting to one of the station operators who originates from Huntly, a power station in NZ. He has an address for me to write to. I need to whip up a CV for him. I have a computer, a printer… and toddlers.

I watch fifty-six people burn at Bradford football stadium, and another thirty-nine get crushed at the European Cup final in Brussels a few weeks later. I don't have anyone to talk to, and as if 1985 hasn't had enough disasters, the *Rainbow Warrior* has been sunk in New Zealand. The clue is in the name Green*peace.* Who on earth wants to bomb a Greenpeace ship?

I don't know what the world is coming to. Do I fancy New Zealand? I should – I never settled in England after living in Australia as a child. We weren't there long, but long enough for me to experience freedom that I was never going to see again.

Jade and Zach are the smartest toddlers – I have a plastic brain, and they can take it apart and fix it together again. They know the names of all the bits. It came with the course, Biology, Brain and Behaviour (SD286). I enrolled before Stan had the Saudi job, but I felt I would manage so I didn't pull out when he went.

I was wrong. Zach has taken to banging his head against the wall to get my attention, Jade takes up a lot of brain bandwidth as I try to outsmart her allergies, and sometimes I lock myself in the loo with a cup of coffee to get myself together. Today I came out partly because my cup is empty but mostly because it is too quiet. The toilet is directly off the kitchen which has never been satisfactory. Jade is laying on the kitchen floor in icy water where the freezer has randomly defrosted. Zach has done a number two on the white lounge carpet and is scrubbing it up with my hairbrush. To top off the total shambles that occurred in the ten minutes I was hiding – a sudden noise diverted my attention from the carpet. An entire nest of kitchen ants has grown wings. They are swarming at the window. The other side of the window are birds, pecking to get at the ants and the noise is horrendous. I didn't even know ants could fly. "Flying ant day" apparently.

Stan comes home on leave, and we have a fabulous holiday in Cornwall at a child-friendly hotel. Jade is a different child in the fresh sea air, but now Stan must go back.

I take him to Gatwick, and on the way home I call in to my GP and tell him I'm pregnant. He doesn't ask about my last period; they had come regularly throughout my pregnancy with Jade, and it isn't yet due. The GP suggested that even if what I claim is true, then the IUD should cause the pregnancy to miscarry. That doesn't sit well with me, so he sends me for a scan, and they remove the IUD, saying it could cause a miscarriage if I *were* pregnant, which they don't believe. I'm better at stating my case this time around.

I phone my tutor to convince her I can't attend the block course. Two toddlers, and pregnant. I have been struggling with the notion of leaving Jade with anyone (volunteers aren't flooding in anyway) and now it has all become too much to cope with.

My tutor tells me my grades are good enough for a waiver for the block course. I can't stop bawling. The course is interesting, with lots of detail about the brain workings behind conditions I have seen in real life. I think it gives me an advantage over the other students. All I have to do is struggle on until the exam in December and make sure I nail it.

Stan's CV that I sent to New Zealand comes back. Tatty is the only way I can describe it. It has been passed around the power stations. They want to know if he can come for an interview. On my way to the library I dump the toddlers at the babyminder and drop a letter in the post-box that explains Stan is in Saudi Arabia and can't pop in for an interview. I borrow the biggest atlas I can find, go home, and sit in the bath and study it. The place with a vacancy has a higher rainfall than Glasgow. I'm not sure about that!

Then… my period doesn't come. Now I *am* scared, and already huge. My GP sends me for a scan at twenty-six weeks. No one can be so big without it being a multiple birth. Strangely a local woman, surprised enough to find she was expecting twins after struggling like myself for her first baby, has delivered triplets.

In my case the scan woman simply repeats, "Oh my, what a huge baby – look at the size of that head."

I can't see. Not that I would have any idea what size a head should be at twenty-six weeks. To be honest, I am a bit disappointed there is only one baby.

27th January 1986

On the *BBC News at Six* I watch sheets of ice cascading from the nose cone of the Challenger as it stands on the launch pad. It was originally planned for launch in July 1985 but there have been a variety of reasons to delay. I think they are desperate now because amongst the payload is the Spartan satellite which will track Halley's comet. Their next opportunity will be in 2061. Becoming more and more uneasy as I watch the footage, I think I *must* act so I dial 192 – Direct Enquiries. It will cost a fortune for the call from the UK to the Kennedy Space Centre in Florida, but I can't *not* phone because I have such a bad feeling. Pregnant, poor, and closed in by snow in Kent, the Space Centre switchboard person tells me there have been several calls from the public, but the engineers believe the launch is safe.

The next afternoon, live on children's TV show *Newsround*, the disaster I predicted unfolds before my eyes.

Dad is babysitting while I collect Stan from Gatwick. I leave home at 2:00 a.m. and skid around the M25, which fortunately is deserted because no one is mad enough to be out on a night like this. It is the coldest month since January 1963 and his plane can't get close to the terminal where the snow is piled up. Stan is dressed in shorts, T shirt and flipflops – what a shock! He reckons I look like a sweet wrapper, but at least I'm warm.

We are going to move to Huntingdonshire in northwest Cambridgeshire, a cheaper area since it doesn't matter where we live if Stan is overseas. We were all supposed to go to Saudi, but his employer has reneged on the deal. Stan thinks I would get arrested over there anyway.

The couple of weeks we have together fly by. Instead of leaving the toddlers with someone, we all head to the airport. I'm thinking the kids are old enough to appreciate an airport, and to be honest even Dad isn't keen on caring for Jade when she's awake.

We cock it up by arriving a day early. It was a fair drive, and I'm not sure they will cope with doing it all over again tomorrow. Stan announces he is giving up the job and staying home. True to his word, the next day goes by and he is still with us. This isn't as simple as it sounds because there is a good chance they will put out a warrant for his arrest. He is under contract. He can *never* go back now, and the New Zealand trail has gone cold as well.

The house is snapped up and at least he can help with the move. We hire a removal van and a driver. At this stage I *should* be able to drive, but I am huge and it's a long way. It is also snowing; the temperature never rises enough to melt the snow. I hate driving on ice.

I wouldn't want to be a solo parent either. For all practical purposes I have been. But he *has* been there, on paper mostly, so I don't feel alone – I can feel the emotional support. Even so, he feels a bit like a spare part now he's home because we have our own systems, like a well-oiled machine. I have even learned to fix things, formerly his superpower.

Cambridgeshire
Stan has found a job at a rubber factory, and I find a new GP. I don't go through my whole saga, but I mention I had been planning to have a home birth. This is something I had insisted on in Kent – not because I have a strong opinion, I just don't want to spend a week under a dripping pipe, and I cannot see a reason to stay at all unless it's to escape Jade, who still wakes up at 3 a.m. and doesn't go back to sleep. However, we are in a rental while we try to work out what to do next and I'm not keen on splattering the place with amniotic fluid. The new GP solemnly promises if I have another hospital birth I won't stay in for a moment longer than I want to, so I agree – but trust me, it's going to be different this time.

1986 has barely begun and it seems like one disaster after another. The Swedish Forsmark nuclear power station detected high levels of radioactivity that isn't coming from Sweden. The wind has been blowing across Europe from the southeast so naturally their eyes turn to Russia.

179

"Nothing to see here," say the Russians. Then: "Maybe a minor accident."

The nuclear fallout is mainly blowing across Scandinavia, but local weather has seen parts of Scotland, Wales and Northern England dumping milk where cows have been eating contaminated grass. There is extensive coverage on the evening news; an accident has occurred at Chernobyl near Kiev sometime within the last five days. Russia has admitted that aid is being sent to Chernobyl but there is no danger elsewhere.

Since radioactivity has been picked up seven hundred miles away, I beg to differ.

I'm weeks overdue once again so my GP gives me a good sweep of the area, and I'm in labour before I reach the car. How come it wasn't that easy before? I'm not in any rush though. We can have dinner and get the toddlers to bed. The neighbour will come over and I plan to be back before they wake up. Perhaps not before Jade wakes up, but I'll try!

It is dark when we eventually leave for the hospital and the contractions are close together. I explain my no drugs, no monitoring policy and the midwife suggests Entonox that I can take or leave. Known as gas and air, it is a mixture of nitrous oxide and oxygen. The other name for it is laughing gas. Stan is immediately drawn to it. By the time the midwife returns roughly an hour later, he is a giggling wreck.

She has a poke about and tells me I am ten centimetres dilated and should be ready to push. But I'm not.

"Don't worry," I tell her. "I am experienced at this – I will know when I should push." The feeling isn't something that can be ignored. Pushing too soon will result in swelling and make things worse. This is a big baby; we know that much already.

She replaces the Entonox tank Stan has drained and gives him her stern look. I had intended to watch TV since the room has one – but Stan is entertainment enough.

About half an hour later she comes back. Stan has laid off the gas and I have been sucking on it; I like the control I have. She takes my blood pressure and her nose wriggles. I spent more than three years *observing*. I know when a nose wriggle isn't a happy one and I demand to know what's wrong.

"Your blood pressure is a bit high, that's all."

Stan grabs her wrist. "She wants to know what it is."

She turns to me and her eyes narrow. "One-ninety over one-twenty."

I do what could be called a sharp intake of breath. "Shit."

"I'm calling your GP," she says and walks swiftly away.

"Oh, Stan, I'm not sure I wanted to know. Now I *am* scared."

There isn't much we can do. I'm not sure if the Entonox could cause my normally low blood pressure to skyrocket or if the labour is doing it and the Entonox relaxing me is preventing things from being worse. Without the midwife to ask, I decide to lay off it. It's close to midnight and I guess my GP is tucked up in bed; he *will* be thrilled.

He comes in wearing a magenta three-piece suit, complete with hot-pink silk shirt and tie. Not the pyjamas I'd imagined. This is not his daytime surgery attire either. He isn't grumpy though. He is worried. My blood pressure *is* too high and given the previous scans he tells the midwife I need to be more than ten centimetres for this baby's head. He believes me when I tell him I will know.

"It needs to be soon," he says.

I know this is code for an upcoming caesarean. I try entering my Zen state. I try to *will* my blood pressure down, rolling over to get on my knees and elbows. I think this is some kind of yoga position. I know nothing about yoga – I don't have the requisite patience – but this position seems like something a yogi would do.

Soon my pink GP is on one side and Stan on the other. I have an arm on each of them, putting my full weight on their shoulders. Both have beads of sweat on their foreheads. Anthony falls onto the bed followed by a ton of amniotic fluid and blood. So much that it rushes along the length of the bed, and splashes over the floor. All I can of think of is the cost of cleaning up if I had done it at home.

Then I remember the placenta; I want a good look – it's the last one. The midwife fetches a kidney dish and the GP rolls his eyes at her. We both know what he means. She disappears and comes back with a plastic washing up bowl. The placenta weighs more than ten pounds by itself and flaps over the edge of the bowl. Anthony is ten pounds five ounces, with a skinny body and giant head. I slide off the soaked bed so it can be cleaned, and they help me onto the scales. I have lost two stone since this afternoon. I start to shake with the shock. The good news is no tear, so no stitches. Stitches down below are the worst thing. And pelvic insufficiency is a rubbish thing.

Part of the attraction of this NHS unit is free disposable nappies. Quite the luxury, especially as I threw so many of the terry nappies out because I'd thrown up over them. But the disposables don't go anywhere near my giant baby, and I take him home wrapped in a hospital towel. On the way we stop at the train station where the florist has just opened, Stan buys two bouquets. Neither of them is for me. One is for the neighbour who stayed and one for the back-up volunteer. Jade has slept all night.

Anthony turns yellow, which clears up quickly in the weak May sun. Suddenly everyone is sleeping all night. Except me. I watch them breathe.

We buy a house. It will have had a thatched roof at one time, and the walls are two feet thick in places. I saw it from the bus, and we were the first people on the doorstep. It needs a huge amount of work, which we aren't scared of, but now New Zealand is sending someone over to interview Stan! My research tells me that you can only emigrate with a maximum of four children to New Zealand. I don't want to go back on the pill, but contraception doesn't seem to work so we save up for a vasectomy – £97.00. Besides, there have been twins in the family; I wouldn't want to have to choose which child to leave behind!

Chapter 22: Emptying Bins

June 6th, 1986 – Space shuttle press conference
I am still upset that I bothered to phone NASA and was
ignored, but now the result of the inquiry is about to be
released so I'm glued to the TV. Seven astronauts died, and
who knows how many onlookers will replay that scene
endlessly in their heads? I know that I already do.

Ever the dramatist, Richard Feynman holds up the press
conference while he calls for a glass of iced water. He places
a rocket booster O-ring into the glass, pulls it out and
demonstrates that it is no longer flexible. Although I did not
know why, I was right – it was the cold that had pushed me to
phone. The O-rings in this context needed to move into and
seal the gap, this is different to a car where the O-ring is a
simple seal already in place. The decision to launch was *not*
supported by all the engineers. Launch day was two degrees
Centigrade, much colder than any other launch. The escape of
hot gas from the failed seal caused the external propellant
tanks to collapse, resulting in a fateful spin on the main shuttle
body and detachment of the boosters. This was just the tip of
the findings; the real problem lay in the mismatch between
NASA management, who estimated shuttle failure due to
engine issues as 1:100,000, and the perception of the engineers
and technicians who put it as low as 1:200.

Kent, January 1987
The clutch has gone on the car, costing £110 which was the
vasectomy money, and the New Zealand interviewer says Stan
doesn't have the right qualifications. It doesn't matter.
Reluctantly I go back on the pill, and he has a job back at the
Centre for Entertainment Games and Bingo. Unfortunately it
is at the Dungeness nuclear power station, which is a three
hour drive on a good day. He has enrolled in an engineering
certificate at Canterbury Technical College; it can't hurt to
upskill.

Initially he comes home at weekends, and my treat on a Friday night is to take Anthony in the pram, order fish and chips then walk to the pub and get a Tuppaware® container filled with Guinness and another with Heineken. One time, while I wait in the pub for the Guinness to settle, I get talking to some bloke. I will talk to anyone. He gives me the phone number of his uncle who is a policeman in New Zealand, I know, the chances of me bumping into him are zero, especially as we aren't going! I lay these containers either side of Ant and collect the fish and chips wrapped in newspaper and plonk the warm package by his feet. Almost alone time.

My efforts of a few minutes solitude at the crack of dawn come crashing down when I hear the toddlers discussing giving Anthony a bath in the kitchen sink. I can hear their IQs banging together coming up with a plan and apart from the danger of the hot tap, or drowning, the idea of the two of them hauling him out of his cot and down two flights of spiral stairs makes me move.

Even with my vigilant parenting, things aren't working. Jade can't bear for Stan to be away, and after a month we move to a beach rental in winter where the beach is halfway up the back door and two of the rooms are flooded. The ice cracks on the kitchen floor when you walk on it in the evenings and the toilet is frozen over every morning, plus we're close to a nuclear power station. We are paying both mortgage and rent so we are poor, but we are together and happy, even though we both think the place is haunted – we regularly hear a child screaming that isn't one of our own.

When I was a young girl – this was one of my favourite places. Miles of golden sand, Roy and I would run flat out without worrying about cutting our feet. We could pull winkles out of their shells with a pin and swallow them. Not anymore. There are signs on the beach, "No children or animals allowed". There is golden stuff oozing up from beneath the sand and if you tread in the wrong place you can be up to your thigh in black sticky stuff that stinks. We put our house in Cambridgeshire up for sale, we haven't even been there a year but we did do a ton of work on the place and it was a bargain when we bought it.

Stan is still studying – his course is all electronics, systems (whatever they are) and maths, plus a communications paper that him and his Dungeness buddies studiously avoid yet *must* pass. So they offer to pay me one pint of Guinness each if I do the required project on their behalf. Thank goodness I have something to put my withering brain into. They have chosen the Chernobyl disaster, and since they work at a nuclear power station they have access to information not released to the public. Inside intel, I love it, and I get 33/35 for an assignment that none of us spent any class time learning how to write. A project like this is much more complex than anything I have had to do with my studies so far and was supposed to be the work of four people, so I am thrilled, three babies and a brain that still works.

One thing that has been intermittently consistent is my bone pain. It disappears the instant that I'm pregnant and reappears within the first few weeks after delivery. But it is getting more frequent. I can't go out without a pushchair to hold onto, and on occasion I have had to crawl around the house with Anthony clenched between my teeth by his clothes. I can't do up the tiny buttons either – my fingers are often blue, even black.

    I am given nifedipine, though as far as I know nifedipine is for high blood pressure. It makes matters much worse, and I cannot stand at all. The next idea is to evoke my potentials. This has to be done in a hospital and involves sticking needles in my legs, thigh and foot, but the needle that is supposed to go into the top of my foot won't work. It needs to hit a nerve and they can't find one. They spent about forty minutes on it before they call the top doctor. He puts the needle in my ankle, and says I am alternately wired – and very brave. Then they shove electric shocks between the two. Apparently there is nothing wrong with me. That's fortunate.

There is something wrong though. The estate agents say the neighbour has piled dirt up against the wall of our Cambridgeshire house covering the damp proof course. He is also throwing things at prospective buyers. After contacting our solicitor, we race up there. We got to know the attached neighbours on the other side after sharing a mouse problem, this side we don't know at all. Not looking for a fight – we arrive with cake. The old lady opens the door and invites us in. Her husband scurries away. She makes tea and we share the cake. Her husband doesn't show himself at all. She explains that she hasn't spoken to him for five years because of his belief that he owns our outside wall. It is the reason the last people left. It *is* unusual in that the wall is part of the boundary. I realise it was such a bargain because it was a problem our solicitor hadn't uncovered when we bought the place.

There is only one thing for it, we bundle him into our van and take him to our solicitor. I guess you *could* call this kidnapping but his wife told him to come with us or don't come home. The solicitor has drawn up a document for the neighbour to sign agreeing that he has no claim over the wall and he will be prosecuted if he continues to pile dirt breaching our damp proof course. It shouldn't be this difficult, he signs, we take him home and leave him to talk to his wife, maybe we saved their marriage.

Hopes I had of returning to work are diminishing – the closures have started. The word asylum means place of safety. Refugees seek asylum. Unfortunately, the asylums built for the mentally ill became dustbins, which is why they came to be known as loony bins. Embarrassing relatives could be dumped and forgotten. How many visitors came to Stone House? I can tell you that for the long-stay wards, a visitor was a rare thing indeed.

Margaret Thatcher's government is intent on emptying the bins. It looks like saving money, which is appreciated by taxpayers who don't understand that community care is expensive. In part, the oil crisis has resulted in belts being tightened and the provision of proper community care has taken a hit. Halfway houses are just smaller dumping grounds, often substandard housing for addicts and not suitable for meaningful recuperation for anyone. There isn't much more on offer unless you have money.

Darenth was cited for closure in 1973, but the task was overwhelming and essentially nothing happened – in fact more facilities opened. A documentary, *Silent Minority* (shown in the UK in 1981), drove a public outcry for the closing of the big asylums for the mentally handicapped. This is not my specialty other than watching the children at play in the grounds of Darenth Park during my nursing training. Over the years there have been snippets in the paper, and the word on the street is that not everyone is happy. Least of all the patients.

I know from my trip to Rampton that people with intellectual disability can be challenging. What I saw there filled me with despair, but what I *didn't* see were nurses bent on neglect and revenge. They were well-motivated people working in desperate conditions, short of staff, resources and support. Recall there had been a similar documentary deriding the care there – *Rampton, The Secret Hospital.* I am not commenting on the lives of the patients, only what I saw.

Over the years intellectual capability and mental health have often been confused. Likewise, the way that people should be treated has changed as perspectives have changed. As early as the 1200s there was the idea of a civic responsibility for the care of people described as *natural idiots.* A Royal Commission in the early 19th century *On Care and Control of The Feeble-Minded* recommended care should be suited to each person's needs and protection should be provided. The outcome didn't match the intent. Care was often brutal and degrading – even physicians of the day maintained poorly mentally equipped souls could withstand cold and hunger admirably well! Isolated colonies or training schools ended up as overcrowded dumping grounds in decrepit buildings.

The move away from these dumping grounds was finally given the impetus it needed in 1984 when the Southwark

187

Mental Handicap Consortium pushed for the re-housing of the Darenth Park patients. They eventually started moving to Southwark in 1986. There were rumblings in the community about the fracturing of relationships as the Darenth Park residents were split up and returned to their area of origin. It must be remembered that some of the residents had been left there as young as three years old. I had a cousin with Down's syndrome who went somewhere, aged four, before I was born.

Those who stepped in to "rescue" the patients held the high ground and were viewed with suspicion not only by the staff on the wards but often also by parents of the residents on the move. This led to poor communication between the agencies and sometimes ended up with people who'd been incompatible on the ward sharing the same small house in the community. The increasing moral turpitude of overworked, shorthanded staff and confused, upset and angry patients led people to breaking point. Anyone might act out when everything they have ever known is thrown into disarray and lifelong friendships are threatened by outsiders. The notion that patients had some kind of relationship with their home patch was tenuous at best. Southwark (and other communities) themselves had changed.

Patients were housed in small groups with people they didn't necessarily like or trust, and staff had to contend with fights within the dwelling. The well-intentioned rescuers were faced with angry neighbours complaining about the noise, and in some cases there was damage to properties on both sides of the fence. The notion that ex-patients could be accepted into the local community were unrealistic. Demoralised staff left. The incoming staff had then lost the link to the original idealism, having never been inside Darenth Park.

The lives of the ex-inpatients, now called *service users,* was enriched in comparison to their lives in the hospital, but they were often bored and lonely, left isolated in the community. I'm not sure that the same thing won't happen for the mentally unwell. They may be better equipped to cope with change but the difference between friends on tap and no friends at all might be one step too far for a lot of them. I'm thinking that the lack of discernible activity surrounding the closure of the asylums for the mentally ill may be because it is easier to wait for the residents to die than to move them.

When contemplating the closure of Stone House, I had already supposed the best nurses would get new jobs (and many from Darenth went to work in Southwark), leaving the most difficult patients with the least able staff. Stone House was also cited for closure, but the number of patients was boosted in 1985 when Mabledon finally shut the doors because its aging Polish community moved in. Natural attrition has seen the numbers at Stone House fall to a hundred and four but some of the last Darenth patients have ended up in villas in the grounds of Stone House. For now, Stone House has a reprieve.

Three babies in four years has left me flabby and tired but it isn't only that – I feel like a waste of space, the waste of oxygen those teachers described on my school report. I do nothing useful. Then Bob Weiland ran the Los Angeles marathon. When I say ran, scuttled would be more accurate, on what can only be described as a tea tray on wheels because he has no legs. He runs using his hands to propel the tea tray to raise money for people worse off than himself. After reading about him I do some deep naval gazing.

Bob lost his legs thanks to a mine in Vietnam but there isn't a shortage of severely disabled people worldwide, many disabled from birth due to drugs containing thalidomide (Distaval and other brands). It was first marketed in 1957 in West Germany as an over-the-counter medication for insomnia and anxiety, and then later for morning sickness in early pregnancy. Mum was offered it when she was pregnant with me (it wasn't withdrawn in the UK until December 1961). There was also a flu treatment called Grippex that contained thalidomide, so not all mothers realised they had taken it. It resulted in many deaths, severe limb deformities, deformed eyes, hearts, alimentary and urinary tracts, blindness and

189

deafness. The drug was never imported into America because Doctor Frances Oldham Kelsey (working for the American FDA) insisted more safety studies should be carried out before the drug was approved there. She saved tens of thousands of lives. There are estimates of some ten thousand *live* babies worldwide being affected (though there could have been easily twice that), with two thousand in the UK alone. Half died within months. There would have been many more that were miscarried or stillborn. Some estimates say 100,000 babies were affected.

I must make the point here that up until the 1960s it was widely believed that nothing could cross the placenta (even though there was no evidence for this belief), and so pregnant women were encouraged to make pregnancy easier upon themselves in whatever way they chose. We now know that this was so far from true, and even following the thalidomide tragedy it took many years for the average GP to really think through the responsibilities they had.

If I am to return to nursing, I need to get fit. On occasion, a sprint or a wrestle is required. My first run is a disaster – I run flat out for about two hundred metres and collapse at the cannon heralding the entry to the local holiday camp. A woman drags her children away, telling them I am drunk. I am deflated and gasping for breath. I need help. But I am not a quitter, and my new plan is to run to one lamp post and walk to the next. Interspersed with the occasional bike ride. I have been running with flat-bottomed silk slipper type shoes. Totally inadequate but the price of running shoes is astronomical!

I started a bucket list when I was seven. Of course I didn't realise what it was then, it was just a list of things I would do – climb Mount Everest, that sort of thing. Over the years things go on my list but often get crossed off. They must be BIG things; everyday wants and wishes do not make the list. I was nineteen when I first heard about a race in Hawaii. The story goes that the competitive spirit between runners and swimmers really started at the finish of the Hawaii perimeter run. Each reckoned they were the fitter but on paper it was Belgian cyclist Eddy Merckx who had tested fittest in terms of oxygen use. No one at the Perimeter race (which was a relay) had cycled the Island's bike race but given that there was a bike race (Around-Oahu Bike Race 115 miles which was raced over two days) and a swimming race (Waikiki rough-water swim over 2.4 miles), as well as the Honolulu marathon (26.219 miles), they felt it would be a great idea to combine the events. The first race in 1978 started with fifteen men. Twelve finished, though they ran out of water for the marathon and the runners had to drink beer! So that went on my list.

I can't swim, at least not any discernible stroke, and I'm struggling to run between two lampposts in one go. My cycling isn't fast, but I have cycled since I was a child, and I have infinite endurance. I have never cycled in any kind of race. I buy some running shoes – Hi-Tec, fucking expensive. They had better work!

With a bit of persistence I can run four kilometres, I prove it to disbelieving Stan by tearing the corner off a poster taped to a lamppost two kilometres away. Still not believing me, he stopped to match the corner on his way to work.

The New Zealand power station people have tracked us down. They have decided that they need Stan after all. What with visas and medicals, it's all going to cost, and we are still paying both mortgage and rent.

It doesn't matter – the immigration department immediately turns us down. Instrument technician is not on the jobs list, and overseas workers can only be brought in where there is a worker shortage. We contact the power station again; Stan is to call himself an engineering technician, but Immigration is unhappy that Zach has had hearing problems, and I have an aberrant reflex in my feet – so they turn us down again. We write a letter requesting reconsideration.

Our rental is going to be used as a summer let for an outrageous price. When the place isn't flooded it will sleep ten people. We can't afford to stay so we move into the local caravan park. The first caravan catches fire. The toddlers are asleep in the double bed, baby Ant in a carrycot in the same room. I smell smoke, rush in, and yell, "Out, now!" I gather Anthony from the cot and the others march out like tin soldiers as the caravan fills with acrid fumes.

We are moved to another caravan and the New Zealand thing is going around and around in my head. They don't even know us. There is a horse running in the Grand National called *Maori Venture*. If it wins, then we *will* make the move happen. If it doesn't then we make our future here. The odds are currently 50:1. We go to put five pounds on it, but the betting shop is closed. It would be irresponsible to put money on a 50:1 outsider when we are broke anyway.

The race is on. We are crowded in the caravan lounge around the tiny TV. Ant is jumping and screaming because the rest of us are jumping and screaming. Ant can't reliably walk – why should he when he has servants. Living in a caravan probably doesn't help, but his brain has forgotten his deficit in the moment. Look at them – so intense – yet they know there isn't any money, only our future on this hopeless nag – but I can see how much it means. I can't let it matter if it wins or if it doesn't.

So many horses fall; *Maori Venture* wins.

Months have passed and we are now in a tent and our campervan. The static caravans were prebooked for the summer-season when we moved in after the beach house was let. We can't put the raised roof (where Zach and Jade sleep) away each day in order to drive, so they cycle a minimum of seven kilometres a day for nursery school. They don't go on the same days (too expensive) so some days they cycle fourteen kilometres. Of course I must run, with the pushchair, fourteen kilometres four days a week.

I have written to the New Zealand Immigration people and told them we can't take the stress; I will run the London Marathon. If I were in New Zealand I intended to run Around the Bays in Auckland, but we can't live like this, and we start looking at properties to buy. The children need a proper home. Immigration responds immediately; they have granted us permanent resident visas. We let the power station know, and they want Stan there to join a small team to commission a new power station, ASAP.

There isn't any financial assistance, and we are penniless. We haven't tried renting the house out because the estate agents keep saying they have buyers that evaporate. Renting it out would be a nightmare anyway, there isn't much work in the area. We rented when we first went there but there are literally hundreds of empty properties, a whole estate of cookie cutter homes so much easier to live in. We make an appointment with the bank manager, our only hope. He peers at us over the top of his reading glasses, his hands pressed flat on the pale-green blotting pad.

"So, you have no funds, an abandoned house miles away that you can't sell, and you want a loan to leave the country which you haven't a hope of repaying because you have both mortgage and rent to pay? Have I got that right?"

It sounds so much worse out loud, and we hadn't even mentioned the neighbour. He rocks back in his huge leather chair, closing his eyes.

"You know what?" He sits upright and looks directly at us. "I *will* do it; it will give me something to talk about at dinner parties for ages! Do not let me down."

Marsden B, we heard your call, see you in the power station village. Our flights are in three weeks.

The Land of The Long White Cloud

October 1987 – November 1996

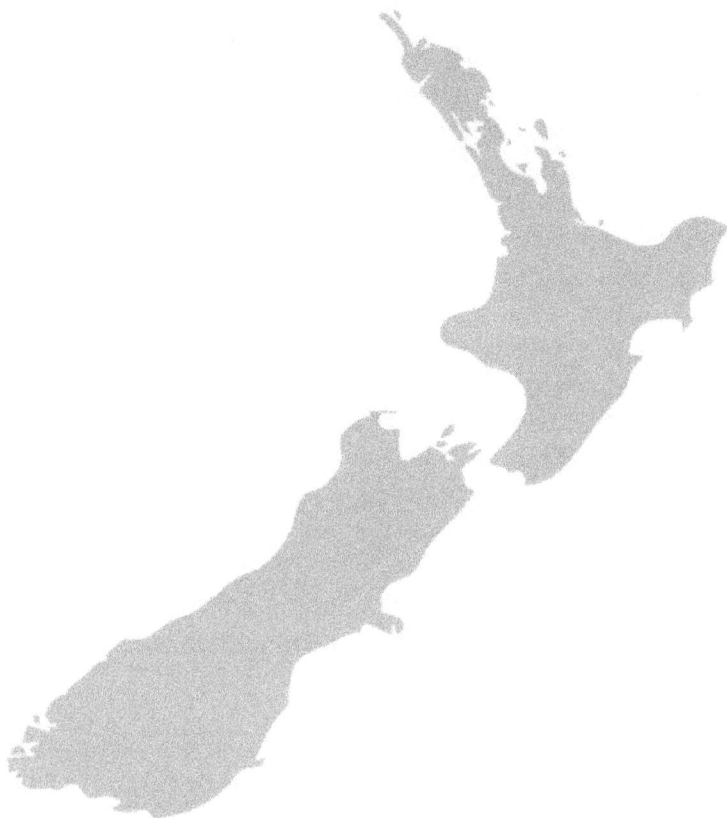

Chapter 23: Flattened

Todd is driving one car, Stan another, since we have double baggage allowance for five people because we are emigrating. We stop at the cash dispenser to empty our account – and the machine sucks the card and returns neither card nor cash. The bank is closed but we can see a light inside. We thump on the massive wooden doors until eventually an employee opens it. They'd had the machine open to restock the money – bad timing, they had no idea of our desperation. It's finally sorted, but now the weather is starting to pack up.

Earlier we had checked the weather report. Michael Fish announced that someone had phoned to say a hurricane was coming, how silly. But the rain is lashing down, we can barely see the car in front, and we are late to the airport. The staff don't have time to check us through, they grab our ton of stuff and run – ours is the last plane to take off before the runways are closed.

Travelling with three children under four – and we meet a couple with four under four – is a nightmare. Even if we hate New Zealand, we are not game for a return journey. We are met in Auckland by a guy who doesn't know why we have come. The project they wanted Stan for isn't going ahead.

We are jetlagged and fall asleep in the temporary bungalow we have been allocated next to the power station dining area. Woken by the afternoon school bus, we can see this community is so poor the children don't even have shoes. Then they feed us pig food for dinner. Mum and Dad had a pig farm before the sweet shop, and they fed pumpkins to their pigs.

We watch the evening news in stunned silence. There are reports of deaths from the storm that hit southeast England as we left. The damage is in glorious technicolour. The caravan site where we lived less than forty-eight hours ago has been turned to matchwood. We would have parked our campervan to protect the tent from the wind. It would have rolled and killed the kids. The devastation is sobering.

Stan is given a job at an aging power station, something he really wouldn't have wanted to do. The first outing for the rest of us is to the local kindergarten. Zach and Jade went to nursery school and I am keen for them to continue. The kindy teacher greets them with a big smile and asks them what they like to do.

"We like to go to the pub," Zach and Jade answer in unison.

What kind of parent do I come across as? I explain that our local pub in the UK had a magician that also made animals out of balloons Tuesday nights and then Punch and Judy on Sunday morning. Jade would be jumping up and down on the BBQ table screaming as Mr. Punch put the baby through the sausage making machine and the sausages came out wrapped in the same material as the baby's clothes. It sounds barbaric but it is true, we will all miss the pub.

There is good news and bad news. The bad news is that there is a waiting list of about a year and Jade will be at the bottom of it. The better news is that they have noticed that Zach struggles to make himself understood. I explain that in the UK he was put on the waiting list for a speech therapist when he was two but never made it to the top. They say they will get someone out here to see him and because he is close to school age, they will enrol him right away to ensure that he has the best start at school.

In England, students start in the September *before* their fifth birthday, so students all start on the same day. Zach would have been four and a half. The school board people chased us to Kent looking for him as I had refused to send him since he couldn't even ask to go to the toilet.

We are shown around the vacant bungalows in the power station village at the end of our first week in temporary accommodation. Naturally we choose the one with a dishwasher. There was a house on the beach but there are some serious drawbacks living on sand. Now we find the estate agents in Cambridgeshire gave the key to someone purporting

196

to be us when they know we are in New Zealand. They have emptied our house, removing even light fittings. Dad has to go and make the wires safe. They have lied to prospective buyers and even tried selling it to someone without an income or money. We are going to have to allow the bank to sell the house to cover the mortgage and loan. We can't afford to keep this up.

For the first six months it seems like a long holiday, we soon work out that we should go to the beach in the morning and bugger the chores because the weather will pack up in the afternoon. I love it. Stan says if he were a girl, he would cry himself to sleep every night. We confirm our original agreement; we will stay for three years even if we both hate it and if we do, we will try Australia. Reasons for leaving the UK remain the same, it is cold and dark, and racism is rampant. We can't afford to go back anyway.

The discussion never comes up again.

I return to nursing as a casual. This doesn't mean my attitude is casual but rather theirs towards me. They will phone when they're desperate. It suits me. The unit is in the same dilapidated state as Mabledon but without a Polish community. It used to be a wooden Victorian villa style building with fancy woodwork around an ample deck and sits in the grounds of the local general hospital. It would have been quite luxurious in its day, but the floor is uneven where the piles are sinking, the linoleum is cracked and has lifted in places, and the windows stick. It's also been poorly repainted several times, so the paint is peeling off.

I know quite a bit about painting because Dad used to make what were then called *picture windows* for extra income. He would take the window out of someone's house on the way home from Hubinuts on a Friday. The new window would be one large sheet of glass, sometimes with casement windows either side, and it always meant at least three or four smaller panes would be removed. He would modify the frame, then give it to Roy and me to sand. He would tell us that a proper job needs elbow grease because if you layer paint over the top of old paint, like the cowboys do, then you are setting the customer up for trouble in the future since the paint will peel. The first time I was phoned for a casual shift Stan was suspicious. So often as a student I was used – put in positions unsafe for me and especially for the patients. My expectation is that they will only call when desperate, and I have visions of being alone and responsible for people I have never met. In fact, I am staff member number six on an evening shift. There is no problem – someone called in sick so I am covering them, and they expect very little from me. One of the older registered nurses seems to think that having me there would be more trouble than I was worth. She softened by the end of the shift.

The project that Stan was called halfway around-the-world for has not eventuated and he is faced with working on the dying days of an aging power station. The only way he can get redundancy is by persuading one of the apprentices to take his role (i.e. by giving the apprentice some of the redundancy money) since his job is not yet technically redundant. Why would we do this? Because we need the year of cheap rent offered in the redundancy package while we come up with a plan. Our plan is to buy a cheap section to live on, and for him to get another job. My job is tenuous but we are managing to get by and the house in Cambridgeshire has finally sold.

I feel like life is replaying my own night-time terrors on live TV. But when no one learns from a disaster it is bound to be repeated, and here we are as the Hillsborough stadium patrons are crushed during the 1989 Liverpool/Notts Forest FA cup semifinal. Ninety-four have died and many hundreds are injured, with a ninety-fifth person dying in hospital a few days later. Has nothing been learned? When there isn't a proper investigation – or even if there is but no learning takes place – we are doomed to repeat things. Sometimes I feel that way myself.

By nature I am someone who goes hunting for work rather than avoid it. I have been called to the ward a few times and it is quite pleasant – much less stress than I expected – so when I am called for a night shift, which I know *will* be short staffed, I'm not unduly worried.

Gail, my offsider, has gone to her midnight "lunch" and I'm reading the paper in the ward office. Lunch is a fair trek through the corridors and down some stairs. The cafeteria isn't open but one of the night porters will sell you some tired meat sandwiches (I found out that meat in this context means tongue) or whatever else is left over from the day.

Out of the corner of my eye I see a shadowy figure run silently past the door. Do I see the glint of a knife?

SHIT, I think I do. I leg after the figure who turns left into the women's dormitory, and now I can see that she – I'm certain this is a female – has the knife in both hands, held high over a sleeping patient. I grab her from behind and the shock sends the knife flying but she lashes out and my glasses go as well, leaving me virtually blind.

I don't have time to search, and without them I have very little chance of finding them. She runs to a bedroom across the corridor, Owen is the only occupant, and since he is deaf and mute he counts as vulnerable, so I follow her. It's still a dumb move on my part even though she is now knife-less.

As I enter, she grabs me, throws me against the wall, punches my face several times with a closed fist, then grabs my shoulders and slams my head against the wall until I fall to the floor in a lifeless heap.

Then nothing.

By the time I come to, Gail is back, and Owen is performing a reenactment for her. Between his wild actions and noises, he demonstrates that he grabbed her from behind and held onto her with all his might until she calmed down. Owen is big but tubby and unfit, and I'm amazed he woke up, being deaf. He demonstrates her swings at me and the banging of my head on the wall.

Gail looks down at me as if to say, *I leave you alone and this is what happens.* Ruby, the knife wielding maniac, has tucked herself up in bed and is pretending to be asleep. Owen is hilarious, and even I smile.

They help me along the corridor back to the office. Gail phones Matron, but of course no one can come and relieve me. I should take myself to the emergency department.

A long walk, especially for someone staggering enough to bounce off the corridor walls. You might think a porter and a wheelchair would be warranted. When I get there, they tell me I must pay.

"Pay for what?" Am I the one not thinking straight? I saved a life in the line of duty, yet I need a chequebook to be given the once over?

"New policy – we can't call someone out in the night for an X-ray unless you are prepared to pay for it."

I'm stony broke, otherwise I wouldn't be taking random shifts and organising three young children. I turn around and stagger back to the MHU. I tell Gail I am OK. She has given Ruby some medication which should at least keep her sedated enough not to leap out of bed looking for a fight with anyone else. Plus, Gail has removed the knives from the kitchen.

By the time morning comes she is doing all the morning stuff while I try and write the notes, but I can't write on the lines. I can't even keep the lines still. I am working way past handover time. Owen busts into the handover and does his routine again. He is so funny (even though the situation isn't) and has all the facial expressions just right. The day shift Charge organises a room in the nurse's home. I clearly can't drive.

When I wake up there is a note shoved under the door.

Go urgently to emergency

I'm not keen, and I'm quite hungry since I skipped breakfast, but a glance in the mirror tells me that all is not well. Even I don't recognise myself! At least my glasses aren't broken; if they had I would be really stuck.

The emergency people tell me that I should not have been expected to pay. I didn't beat myself up and accidents never warrant a charge. They think I am OK, but I'm to take a few days off. Since I'm a casual that just means I don't get paid. If I didn't like falling out of a train, then I don't like this even more. I drive home and Stan is angry when he sees the mess.

I promised to help with the can collection for the childcare centre fundraiser. I can't weigh the cans and work out the cash, so I do the crushing. The next day I doze all day. I feel like I have been run over by a bus. This year I enrolled in Organic and Biological Chemistry via Massey University; I have decided to be a biochemist in deference to the bucket list. A head injury isn't going to help at all.

The following day I get a phone call. The hospital needs someone to escort a patient to a secure unit. They can't tell me who it is – they are only the person who does the organising – but it will be by ambulance, and money for old rope since the patient will be sedated and I will be paid for a full shift. It isn't as great as it sounds because it will take a whole shift by my estimation. They want me at the afternoon handover. I'm torn, but broke, between a rock and a hard place.

Everyone stares as I walk through the office door. I can hear sharp intakes of breath. I know I look horrific – my black eyes are half closed, my nose is bent, and my cheeks are shades of yellow, green, purple and blue. In fact, I would be unrecognisable to most people if not for my hair. The psychiatrist who'd tried to maintain there was nothing wrong with the woman who'd attempted to stab someone in the night and beat me half to death – is visibly surprised and realises that he has zero legs to stand on. Metaphorically speaking. The staff had spent the past three days trying to convince him that she needed more intensive care than an open ward could offer, and he had been recalcitrant. I am the one to do the escort, though she should have already gone for the safety of everyone.

At least Ruby is *very* apologetic when she sees the state of me. She isn't sedated, or not so it shows, but so very sorry. She attempts to make the journey the best it could be under the circumstances by some pleasant chatter about families and stuff. We get the full ambulance treatment, sirens and everything – they have been told that the sedation is not to wear off or I could be trapped in the back of an ambulance with a mad woman! I have a little bag with an emergency injection, though I am not sure how that would work; I would be as likely to stab myself in a fight!

The secure unit staff are staggered at the state of me. She is well known to them, though they wouldn't have anticipated such violence. Since neither Ruby nor her family were objecting to the transfer, how had she been left for so long on an open ward? I have never been in the position of accompanying someone who has the capacity to become volatile before, but the ambulance guys are great, and we *are* back in less than the whole shift. It is dark though, and while I'm driving home with my eyes still half closed I realise I couldn't have worked a shift – even doing nothing for seven hours has totally worn me out.

There hasn't been any kind of investigation, and no one has asked me anything. Unexpectedly I am asked if I would take on Thursday and Friday nights each week as a permanent staff member. I don't have to debate for long because Friday night is mostly Saturday, and I will get penal rates.

Stan has a new job with a different outfit and with my now guaranteed income we are finally able to buy a small section within walking distance of the village that opened its arms to us. I am the one to hammer the first post into the newly scraped ground on New Years Day in 1990. We are to become part-time builders. We can't get a mortgage for a dwelling because we don't have a credit rating.

I have the block course for my latest university paper. I am quite organised these days and everything is going well. The lab work is assessed by a repetition of one of the labs with *unknowns*. We aren't told which lab practical it will be until the night before. We must pass it to succeed, even if we get 100% for everything else in the course.

On Thursday, the day before our assessment, I am so ill I cannot get to the lab; I have diarrhoea that won't stop. It is like something we all had a few months ago. I phone the course controller, who tries hard to persuade me to attend. He probably thinks I was out on the turps last night, but I have had my head down studying hard. I want to lift my grades, and I'm enjoying this paper. I think I have found my true vocation.

Thursday afternoon the news seeps out: the experiment we are to do for our test tomorrow is the experiment to determine the saponification value and iodine value of an unknown fatty acid. The class did it this morning and I didn't.

I am up late; I write the experiment up tidily, leaving gaps for weights and values so I know exactly what I'm doing and don't miss out any steps and I get the maths correct. I write it like a guide for idiots. The calculations will be my Achilles heel and I have no idea how to carry out what I have said I will do.

The lab practical is under test conditions – individual work, no conferring. Everyone looks organised as we are each given our mystery lipid. The saponification value will give me an estimate of how long the carbon chain is. Iodine value will tell me how many double bonds it has. I am perplexed because the average chain length seems to be too long to be lard or butter, but the iodine value says there are no double bonds, which rules out oils.

I assume that I have somehow cocked it up but I dutifully document everything I have done. I check the calculations, and my best guess is coconut fat because I can't think of anything else. I'm astonished when I turn out to be right. The course controller is impressed; he said he tried so hard to persuade me to turn up yesterday because he knew that missing the practice was going to make it almost impossible for me to pass. He says he will be looking out for my name in the future. There is also a definite upwards trend in my grades.

Additionally, things are looking better on the home front. We are getting a little advance from the bank for every bit of value that we add to the property. We have hand built every downstairs wall, with Stan leaving a cutting list, me cutting nogs and studs all day, then in the evenings we have been nailing everything together producing the next wall. It's true that sometimes our walls aren't right and have to come down. The latest advance from the bank has given us enough money to get the upstairs walls delivered pre-built which will speed things up considerably. I can see a time when we will move out of the dodgy caravan. We have to ply the roof with water during the day because we can smell the frame turning to charcoal. We have already been in one caravan that caught fire. If I were to tear back a little of the lining to check it, oxygen could seep in and precipitate a fire. I will definitely tear it to see when we move into the house. The caravan will be going to the tip. If someone less diligent at cooling it were to have it and it caught fire, how would I feel then?

Chapter 24: Fading Away

I have a concern closer to home. Anthony is wasting away. In the first couple of years he grew in line with that expected of a giant baby. He was 4.68 kg at birth and is 16 kg now. But his trajectory dropped away, and he hasn't gained *any* weight in the last year. He is also tired all the time. I have been so concerned that the children have moved into the unfinished house to sleep because it is drier. Warm water comes in the form of filled black bin bags left all day in what passes for a front garden (bare sand littered with building materials). Once the sun has made it warm or at least tepid, we put it into a fish bin to bath the kids. Many children have worse, but now things have gone downhill even further.

Stan's Dad has died unexpectedly. I say unexpectedly because he was going to die from bowel, stomach and lung cancer, but in fact he departed hastily due to an undiagnosed aortic aneurysm that burst on the operating table.

As is common amongst his generation, his was the only name on the rent book; the bank account, and the utilities. Mum, penniless and bereaved, had a letter threatening to cut off the power.

We had the chat with the kids about Granddad being dead. They know what dead means. We held a wake at the local club; loads of people came and we had a great time. He was at least spared the ravages of a lingering death from cancer; this gave us some consolation and we have moved on.

Not so for Lil, she has always been tiny but now she has lost a significant amount of weight and is not recovering from her grief. Inexplicably she decides to travel alone, via a cargo plane out of Luton to stay with us. There is, of course, an open invitation but the timing isn't great. We don't have hot water, the power is illegally run from a builder's pole and the walls are not insulated or lined. On the plus side, the windows are in and we have a roof.

Everything has gone to plan – until we try and leave the airport. Ant won't leave. He refuses to budge because he is waiting for Granddad. I take him aside and remind him of the chat that we had about being dead which he assures me he got, but why has Grandma not bought him with her? I am temporarily speechless, but he won't waver, he is waiting until Granddad comes and he won't be talked out of it. I try and get Mum to talk to him, but she won't. I can see that she is all in from the travel, she doesn't look at all well. She doesn't want to explain to a five-year-old what she has done with Granddad. We literally carry him kicking and screaming from the airport with the whole world watching on. I know they are silently suspecting child abuse, and he makes an awful scene trying to strap him into the car seat.

My GP has run out of ideas about Ant's failure to gain weight and organises an appointment with the hospital paediatrician. But when we get there the specialist takes one look at the strapping, healthy older children and suggests I have too much on my hands – perhaps I don't realise that Anthony isn't getting properly fed. I am wondering now if an incident last summer with the gambling people hasn't been put right.

When they phoned me I thought they wanted a donation, but that wasn't it. Then I thought it was a survey. But it wasn't. They'd called because they'd been told about my *gambling problem.* They had been led to believe it resulted in my children not getting afternoon tea.

Firstly, afternoon tea is a nice to have, not an essential meal. Secondly, if we win any money at the races Ant and I have afternoon tea to celebrate and then have afternoon tea *again* when we get Zach and Jade from the school bus. Thirdly, I spend the princely sum of six dollars every six weeks at the racetrack, which is only open for part of the year. We are in credit anyway after winning a hundred and ten dollars for a one dollar bet. I was so surprised I double-checked with the girlie on the counter in case she had to make good on missing money – the place runs on volunteers after all.

Not being burdened by knowledge, Ant and I have a great strategy; we bet on the grey, and if there isn't a grey then we bet on the rider with the loudest shirt, or the horse that has pooed most recently. We think that will give the horse a boost! I am literally at the racecourse with a small boy looking for a horse in the act of having a poo. Ant thinks it's hilarious, and yet the Gambler's Anonymous lady suggested that horse racing wasn't an ideal outing for a child!

It shows how careful you have to be though – who is watching and listening?

Perhaps I am on some kind of bad mother list. Since it is wrong to hit people, I gather my offspring and leave the paediatrician to write whatever he likes. I need to find a proper doctor for Anthony – one who will listen.

Things aren't great at home either, Ant and Lil argue every day. The children have been trained to wash their cup and put it away even if it was only water they had. Ant comes complaining "She's doing it ALL wrong."

"What's wrong sweetheart?"

"It's Nan –, she says I can't wash up but she is leaving the cup on the bench, people will get sick."

It's true that meningitis warnings have been all over the TV. Lil joins in.

"You can't expect a five-year-old to wash up properly."

It is evident that Ant is sick, and Lil is wracked with grief – I need to cut them both some slack, but refereeing fights between a five-year-old and a pensioner is wearing me down.

—∿—

It's late but I have been called back to work for an extra night. A pain but as it's a Saturday it is penal rates all night, so I can hardly refuse. We practically went straight out to harriers when I got home this morning. We all run. Not Stan so much, though on occasion he has. His forte is archery, and often we rush from one event to another. After harriers we had supermarket shopping, so I had no chance for a nap. When it gets too late – I stay awake rather than bugger up the next night's sleep, but now they need me to babysit a woman in a coma. It's technically not my job since she's on a medical ward, but because she is known to the mental health team – they want me there.

Before I arrive in time for the overnight shift she has livened up and somehow removed the tap from the radiator in her room and flooded the place. That will be because there wasn't anyone sitting with her. It is going to be a long night.

She has diabetes. This is the type two diabetes that was glossed over during my training as being uncommon. The incidence is rising alarmingly worldwide. Driven by modern life, apparently. This woman is unpleasant at the best of times, and her blood glucose levels are so high she should still be in a coma. Instead, she is causing mayhem.

A diabetic coma can occur because blood glucose levels are very low or high; an emergency is considered lower than 2.8 mmol or more than 13.5 mmol of glucose per litre of blood (though I have known nurses to regularly test higher than that at work). The Americans, of course, use a totally different measurement of mg per decilitre. Not only is a decilitre not an SI unit (Système International d'Unités, the best thing to come out of France), but it confuses the hell out of people. A millimole is one thousandth of a mole; a mole is 602 hexillion molecules of anything, but in this case glucose. The American system relies on the weight (mass actually) of glucose in one hundred millilitres (100 mL) of blood. This woman's coma is the result of extremely high levels of glucose, 29 mmol per litre (in US units this equates to 522.5 mg per 100 mL). Ordinarily between meals (since she has been in a coma she hasn't eaten), you would expect 4–7 mmol per litre (72–126 mg per 100 mL).

She is a big and intimidating woman who's on a medical ward because her problems are life-threatening but now she could be said to be threatening the lives of others. Will the MHU take her? "Hell no."

No surprise there; I told the doctor it wouldn't happen when he suggested it. On night shift in the MHU, the staff are the most experienced on the unit. In mental health. All are psych registered, not general, and no one should have the complexity of this medical event thrust upon them however badly she is behaving.

I make her a cup of tea. Which works. For a while.

This diabetic lady has a tentative diagnosis of bipolar disorder or borderline personality disorder. She uses her diabetes for attention. I have heard of people purposefully putting themselves at risk to get out of a situation they are unhappy about – for instance, sinking into a diabetic coma in police custody. It sounds nuts to me.

Ruby – the woman who beat me up – has full-on bipolar disorder, previously called manic depression. I have met many and for the most part these are delightful people – funny, charismatic, often smart and talented, and on occasion barely able to move, gripped with a severe depression draining their world of colour.

Bipolar disorder is treatable, or at least manageable, but currently most people are of the view that personality disorder is not. To the extent that in the UK, section 136, used by police to uplift persons believed to be a danger to themselves or others, also talks about adding *and amenable to treatment.* Those deemed not to be amenable to treatment then end up in a police cell rather than a hospital.

My own experience of people with any personality disorder has been negative. I'm not going to describe the people I have met. I truly don't want to dwell on any of them. Those who wind up in hospital are often women diagnosed with borderline personality disorder. Men with psychopathic or sociopathic tendencies might be high-functioning businessmen, serial killers or similar. The women have a tendency to live their lives as if they are the central character in a bad soap opera. I'm generalising of course, some men can be exactly as manipulative. The damage to loved ones can be immense. I am not convinced people choose to live their lives this way. Many patients have been damaged by childhood abuse and simply can't seem to get on top of life. A few manage to escape, requiring massive input from too few psychologists, but dealing with them on a day-to-day basis is demoralising and exhausting. They are likely to end up losing access to their children and damaging themselves with repeated drug overdoses – generally prescription drugs which have never done anything useful for them anyway. Ultimately, nobody wins.

If we return to the business of being *amenable to treatment* and look at the extreme end of the personality disorders, to the psychopaths and potential serial killers of the world, there must have been a time before they committed a crime they could be incarcerated for, and there will be a time when they need to be released for those who *have* committed such a crime. What then? If psychiatrists will only take on treatable patients? Many of the long-stay patients I met during my training have been irreparably damaged by past treatment, so this can't be an across-the-board stance; it only applies to dangerous people, those who not only do not want to be treated, but whom the medics' view is they can't be treated. We are treading on very dodgy ground if we say they should be locked in prison *in case* they commit a felony. I wish I knew what the answer is, but I don't.

—◊—

Lil refused to go home within the time frame of her return ticket but now the UK government have threatened to stop her pension. Our task here is done, she has gained weight, got involved with the local fifties forward group and made friends so we are sending her back in much better shape than she arrived.

Anthony was so tired at Christmas that he went back to bed rather than open his presents, but I have had some luck with another GP. She is Vietnamese, she listens, and she persists. The ultimate diagnosis has taken us by surprise since it turns out we are *all* sick! Last year was especially good for the family in a sporting sense, making it even harder to fathom. I ran two marathons, my first in a time of 3:48:52, and the weather was appalling, I had to be heated up in the medical tent. Anyone who knows about running will know that this is a decent pace for a first timer. My bone pain isn't affected by running, but sometimes the pain prevents a run. Stan has done especially well in his archery tournaments and the offspring have all excelled in cross country.

Now we have all been diagnosed with giardiasis. I recall the night that everyone was so sick we ended up dragging our bedding into the hallway outside the loo. That was at least eighteen months ago, and it accounts for the near disaster at the block course last year. The lab lady at the hospital was so excited – she had never seen it before.

When we were first ill, Stan and I blamed the sausage sizzle the kids had queued up for after my first half marathon. Neither of us realised they were getting their sausages and immediately joining the end of the queue for more. But that night the toll of washing vomit off their sheets had me slinging them straight in the bath, with Stan and me succumbing an hour or so later. He did have a couple of sausages, but I have never been one for dodgy food. I even told our GP I thought it was giardia, but he pooh-poohed me. The rest of us recovered. Well, sort of. Zach was the only one who seemed fully recovered and the lab lady said he had the worst infestation; she said new cysts were hatching every few weeks. None of us have managed to eradicate it. My only other idea would be that I picked it up from a forest tramp. I am usually very careful, I don't recall drinking from a stream but could have washed my dishes, or even my toothbrush. Medically – dodgy water is more likely.

The treatment, we are assured, is simple. A course of metronidazole. The others are OK. I am much worse because the metronidazole has resulted in intestinal thrush, and the treatment is a month's worth of horse pills. On night shift I am sliding off my chair as my blood glucose and blood pressure falls into my boots. I'm certain I am going to die. I don't.

—◠◡◠—

Back in the UK, the Friern finally closed on 1 April 1993. April Fool's Day. On 31 March managerial types were still rushing around trying to accommodate the remaining patients.

Ten years' notice was insufficient, it seems. It marks the end of the Victorian legacy.

In pre-Georgian times people incapacitated by lunacy or feeblemindedness lived with their families. If they had none then they walked the highways and byways with other social outcasts or ended up in jail or the workhouse. The oldest workhouses date back to the mid-1600s, but gradually, housing lunatics became a lucrative business. By 1800 there were around two thousand lunatics in small homes dotted across England. Many were private homes, with others run by church parishes. Some not so bad and some appalling. There were only a few hospitals catering to two or three hundred people at the most and offering dubious care.

Mental health status was helped by the madness of King George III. He first became ill in 1765 (probably porphyria or possibly bipolar disorder), but it was temporary and kept hidden even from Queen Charlotte. By the turn of the century, he was placed under her guardianship and George IV was appointed Prince Regent since his father had become unable to rule. George IV was king in his own right for ten years and died childless, so the throne passed to his next brother William. William IV only lasted seven years, and since he was without legitimate children his niece Victoria became Queen aged eighteen in 1837. County asylums had already been recommended in 1807, financed by the poor rates, but when reformist John Connolly visited establishments in the 1830s, he found cold, shackled, near naked patients with beds of straw and a pestilent air at the hands of often cruel and brutal keepers. He doubted the ability of those driven by money to recognise insanity or provide treatment. County asylums became mandatory by 1845, resulting in the period of Victorian asylums that housed over 100,000 mentally ill people by the end of the century.

Of the asylums in existence by the middle 1800s, almost all of them declared that restraints would no longer be used. Moral care was the order of the day. The Friern (then Colney Hatch) was built for 1250 inmates. Even before it opened in 1851 this number was considered too many for the aspirations of the time. There were 2,000 within ten years and the good intentions fell by the wayside due to overcrowding and the admission of paupers who were deemed unsuited to luxuries (as a pauper myself I have always been keen on a bit of luxury). Restraints had come back in use by 1861. Degenerates and defectives were now imprisoned.

A lunatic's lot didn't really improve until the 1930 Mental Health Act introduced the notion of voluntary patients and outpatients. This was anticipated to reduce the number of patients. The paying mentally ill could vote with their feet, but numbers kept rising. By 1937 the Friern housed 2,700 people and a lot of them had untreatable conditions that produced psychiatric symptoms: brain tumours, metabolic syndromes and lead poisoning, and notably syphilis which leads to GPI that Wilf had, commonly termed paralysis. Plus, there were victims of WWI. In the UK 80,000 cases of war neurosis were diagnosed, commonly known as shell shock, but many more were hospitalised as paupers having failed to meet the criteria for a war victim.

I hadn't realised that those on social security still got payments even when they were hospitalised long term. These costs together with the cost of building maintenance, plus the idealism of the 1960s and effectiveness of new medication, gave the appearance that custodial care was somehow ethically wonky. The various documentaries cemented a grim story in the eyes of the public, so the stars were aligned for the emptying of the bins to continue at an increased pace. The value of the buildings and land only added to the reasons to close.

The last months of the Friern were exactly as I had supposed they would be – the most talented staff left first, resources disappeared to community care homes, and the easiest patients to move were first out. This left staff at the edge of retirement, those with dubious qualities, and overworked agency staff to look after the neediest patients in the worst conditions.

What is misunderstood is that the average person has their own institutions to support their wellbeing. Their workplace, school, university, swimming club, gym, art class etc. People have somewhere to be and social contacts to enrich their lives. Not many sit alone in rooms, frequently lacking the comforts most take for granted – often cold because heating is expensive, possibly without even a TV for companionship. The community isn't flocking to embrace the discharged mentally ill, and adequate community support is a fairytale. This isn't just a UK problem; all over the world asylums are closing. Kingseat and Tokanui are on the chopping block, Carrington is closing this year. Their days are done.

Yet ex-patients are expected to manage themselves under these circumstances. Good luck with that!

It's going to be a grim nightshift tonight; I've been told my offsider has been killed in a car crash. No idea who I will be working with.

Chapter 25: Firefighting

The reality is that my education has come to a halt. On nightshift I try to get as much done as I can, and I have completed every extramural paper that remotely interests me. Now I must change my subject or quit. I have almost two years of full-time study to complete a biochemistry degree, and it can only be done as an internal student. I would have to show up to class and do lab stuff all year, not just block courses. Not only do we need my wage to pay the bills, but for me to live halfway across the country would cost even more money. As usual, we don't have savings.

I'm restless. My friends say either I go now, or I will never come back to it and my chance will have vaporised. The children are eleven, ten and eight. People say I should go before they are teenagers when they will really need me. Two years though. I could probably squash it into eighteen months. I would have to work as well, to pay for accommodation and food, even if I lived on cardboard.

In the end I broach the subject at work. They could agree to six months' unpaid leave now, and six months at the end of next year. Is it doable? It wouldn't be the whole six months – the student semester is shorter. Is it possible to cram two years' full-time study into one? The happy professor thinks so. I would still need a job.

The university runs in semesters – almost. With one of the papers I would have to do the theory for it by myself and the lab work on my return next year. There will be class clashes, possibly exam clashes, but they have faith in my talent to make it work. Unfortunately the student funding people don't allow for one semester of study – I have to do a full year of papers to get any help from them. So I enrol for a full year of study that can't possibly be undertaken in one semester and worry about how it will pan out while I am there. I get accommodation in the nurses' home – contacts count for something. It still costs.

215

I hadn't banked on the homesickness. The professor with the faith would pick up the tissue box every time I knocked on his door. I ate baked potato every night and gave up tea to save money on tea bags. I took my pushbike for transport and got a job with the Red Cross – an old lady with a broken back and no one to turn her in the night. She needed putting to bed as late as possible and getting out of bed and showered as early as possible. Which suited me as I studied every minute except Thursday evenings when I read my *New Scientist* with a happy hour half-price pint of Guinness. Treat day, although the Guinness was in lieu of dinner. Between freezing and crying, I got through.

—⟋⟍⟋⟍—

Half the MHU has been taken away. Literally – jacked up, put on the back of a truck and gone! It hasn't gone far but it marks the start of the exciting new build. We have been poring over colours and materials for months, staff and long-term or repeat customers, even visitors. But meanwhile the loss of a building means we have half the beds and are bursting at the seams.

It is also unusual that we have a woman with Down's syndrome on the ward. She is classed as elderly at forty-seven and has dementia – not something we are ideally equipped to deal with. Though the Aged Care Unit isn't right for someone young and mobile either. This must be a scary place for someone intellectually disabled and further impaired by dementia. With family issues to deal with, someone has to offer a place of safety for this woman.

There is also Mary, currently a *very* regular customer. Clearly distressed, she has continuously sought admission for a variety of reasons that no one has got to the bottom of. Wanting to be in a run-down MHU with strange bedfellows rather than a perfectly decent home and a seemingly a loving family simply doesn't make sense. She has, however, worn out two psychiatrists and all the ward staff. I must admit to being downcast to find both ladies here when there are already enough acutely disturbed people, and a door we are not, by law, allowed to lock (the gazetted locked ward having been trucked away). As usual we have only two staff; me and new graduate Janine, and no one nearby to call on.

We are stretched from the start. Our lady with Down's syndrome can't stop wandering, she has no idea where she is or where her family has gone. Whatever we say or do, it doesn't help her. She can't tie both of us up either, since the lady who always wants to be here is now demanding to leave. We are on a sticky wicket, morally we can't allow someone to leave in the night and yet we have no mandate to hold onto anyone. They can all leave if they so desire. We plough on, getting most people settled into bed, and eventually are left only with the lady who wants to leave. She has exhausted our patience – not only tonight but over the last year. We *are* entitled to a meal break, but it isn't looking likely. Usually, one person will go off the ward and leave the other in sole charge. This is a situation that has perpetuated for years, and we are told it is a luxury to have two staff overnight. On so many levels this is wrong and has been proven to be wrong, I was alone when I got beaten half to death saving someone from a knife attack, but nothing changes.

Suddenly, and rather dramatically, a fistful of firefighters burst through the door, head to toe in full-on fighting gear complete with breathing apparatus. Apparently the locked ward is on fire. I explain how it is on the back of a truck and elsewhere so unlikely to be on fire. I am not making any headway. It has come up on their alarm system, which is quite interesting because there won't be any power to it, yet the fire station is getting a signal.

The commotion has already started to wake a few people. I try to get the firefighters to leave – they refuse. They MUST check, despite my protests, because they believe there *is* a fire somewhere.

I am required to show them around. This old unit doesn't have individual bedrooms, but small dormitories, the smallest being four beds with curtains around each bed. They want to pull back each curtain and check for fire and so they wake up a dozen or so psychotic patients plus the lady with Down's we only just got to sleep.

We may as well have set off the alarm and then we could have made the excuse it was a fire drill and everyone could have had a lie-in as a reward for being so calm and efficient, but instead we have a situation where patients believe spacemen have arrived. They are fuelling the story between them, and things are getting seriously out of hand. The firemen can't find a fire and depart, leaving us in a state not far short of chaos.

Janine and I make heaps of cocoa, give out prn (as necessary) medication to those who think the spacemen have come to take them for anal probing, and we try very hard to convince them the fire brigade is just doing their job. Our lady with Down's keeps screaming and some of the motherly types are trying to calm her, while Janine tries ringing for help but everywhere is short because it is lunchtime (between 1 a.m. and 2 a.m.). Gradually everyone gets back in bed but there is an empty bed and my heart sinks. We have lost the woman who has spent so much of her recent life trying to get admitted.

"It's OK," Janine tells me. "She was making such a fuss – I got her to sign a discharge against advice form. We did our best."

Really, we did. We notify Matron, complain we haven't been relieved for lunch, and say we don't feel one person should be left here alone. We are ignored as usual. We do not inform the police or phone her husband because we have no sense she is in any particular danger. They are all sick of trailing around after her. We *should* have informed everyone.

When I think about her, I realise she reminds me so much of my neighbour's mother from years ago who drove everyone completely mad with her continuous handwringing and wailing. Initially you are full of care and concern until you realise it isn't helping anyone, and you are getting stressed yourself. The neighbour's mother was vastly improved by a leucotomy, an operation to sever the connections between each hemisphere of her brain. The word comes from the Greek for "cutting white", which in this case refers to the white

218

matter of the brain. Even back in the early eighties it was an old-fashioned treatment from a position of desperation. There is not a chance it would be considered in the 1990s.

The next day I found that she went home and hung herself. In her pocket was a note with a list of things that she could do. One of the items on the list was *sneak away and hang yourself.* A leucotomy may have saved her life.

Naturally I am waiting for the enquiry. I was, after all, the person in charge.

—∿—

Not long afterwards we have a newcomer. We are still in the same half a unit, short of space and not gazetted for door locking. I work Monday and Tuesday day shift on a regular basis, so I have come across most people during the daytime at some stage, and most are returning customers. This guy is already asleep when we arrive for our Friday nightshift. He has been admitted for depression. The dayshift reckon he is fine and won't be a problem. I'm not happy to be responsible for someone I have never met, but no one wants to be woken up just to be introduced to new staff. I am conflicted but capitulate.

Things seem pretty settled. Work has started on the build. The builders left a digger outside with the keys in. I saw it on the way in and took the keys because the first thing I thought of when I saw it was how much fun it would be to nick a digger – I was tempted myself! There are several young men here who, for certain, would think it was a jolly jape. In fact, we have an experienced driver of such machinery; he got admitted because he drove a digger up onto a pile of logs and no one can get it down.

I am with Alma tonight. She is funny, another casual. Since the car crash that took my partner there have been a string of casual nurses. Usually they at least volunteer; anyone who doesn't want to do mental health shouldn't. Being with someone too terrified to move is worse than being alone. Even a voluntary nurse isn't always OK. We had a new graduate here one time whose heart was set on mental health. Everything appeared to be going well until there was a fight in the kitchen. I entered in time for a hurtling body to smack my hand into the wall and break my thumb. The new grad sped past the open door, so I imagined she had gone for help – good thinking. That wasn't what happened. She had gone to the linen room to cry and never came back. Last I heard she got a job as an industrial nurse. You can get through your training without ever encountering a fight, and until you do you can't know how you will react. Alma and I are happy to be working together.

Everyone is tucked up; I start on a letter I have been meaning to write and Alma has her knitting out. It isn't too hard to stay awake on a cruisy night until after lunch or whatever it is you call eating at 1:00 a.m. You can check all the beds, make cocoa for anyone who wakes – early wakening is common – but if everyone is asleep most staff start to struggle by 3:00 am. I make a family newspaper for our various relatives so I can stay awake. I get the kids to write stuff, and I put together race results for all of us – that sort of thing. I don't approve of staff who push a couple of armchairs together and curl up under a blanket. Not really the coiled spring, ready to react to an emergency. I guess it matters less in some circumstances.

We are approaching those difficult hours when the new guy surfaces. He seems agitated. I offer him the chance to sit and chat, but he is pacing and mumbling in front of the unlocked door. I don't know him – no one really does. He had the usual interview with the psychiatrist on duty which may or may not be someone who has seen him before, but there aren't proper notes – just a one-page handwritten summary that is difficult to read and talks of him feeling down and waking early but he denies feeling suicidal. It is hard to fathom why he has been admitted given the scarcity of beds. The level of acuity required for admission has been higher than average recently. I'm not happy. I get between him and the door trying to cajole him back to bed, but he isn't having any of it and doesn't want to chat. After the best part of thirty minutes he comes right out with it – he wants to leave.

The last woman who left hung herself and there is something making me concerned about this guy. We have at least three hours before the day shift is due. Can two of us hold onto one bloke without doing anything illegal?

No – turns out to be the answer. I end up blocking the door... for three hours. Alma has tried to get help – even a male orderly might have been able to do something useful – but as usual our needs are not hospital priority. I succeed in preventing him from leaving and eventually he gives up and slides back into bed not long before the day shift arrives. I write on his notes in capital letters that I believe he is actively suicidal. I write on the main sheet that I prevented him from leaving because I felt I had no choice.

After I left for home, the day shift let him go for a walk. He took a dive off the ambulance bridge and died in A&E after his brain stem coned (the brain is forced through a small opening at the base of the skull where it meets the spinal cord, like a hernia of the brain).

Nothing happens. Why should I have expected anything different? Who on earth would talk to me? No one has *ever* asked me anything when something bad has gone down. I am invisible.

I'd tried to prepare for the homesickness, but I didn't prepare for the train derailment. I had taken sleeping tablets for the overnight train and didn't notice the train coming off the tracks. Someone was shining a flashlight in my eyes, telling me to get off; the train was on a clear slant. Initially I fell straight back to sleep, thinking I was dreaming. But flashlight guy saw me on his way back and helped me off. In the distance were bright lights, and the passengers waiting for buses. Then the bus broke down. By now I have some good friends who make my life better.

I've only been gone five weeks when Stan turns up unexpectedly for my birthday. I say unexpected – I knew something was afoot. My friends were almost bullying me about where I would be for the weekend (I just wanted to curl up and rock), so of course they were all in on it.

We have a family holiday in September – skiing on a live volcano. Jade wrote a will leaving everything to her friend – I hope that doesn't include her dog. The temperature of the crater lake has been rising – it's been all over the news. The volcano blew the following week, the ash carpeted the university quad. Being so close to finishing, I *have* to make it through.

In the end Stan put Jade on a train and sent her to Palmerston North, much like a package. He says she's moody and he's panicked that it could be her periods about to start, and although a brilliant father – he doesn't feel up to those kinds of issues. She has a room next to mine in the nurses' home – so grown up.

You *know* when you have passed your exams, so I knew I had my BSc in biochemistry and molecular biology, but I felt as though my right arm had been cut off. Jade skipped across the quad to the exam room as I exited. We had the overnight train booked so went for an early celebration at Pizza Hut. Unbeknown to me, Jade filled her bag with Smarties. No one got any sleep that night – maybe not so grown-up after all.

The last event of the year is Stan's fortieth birthday. We have a party, in our house! It looks finished from the outside (if you ignore the bombsite of a garden). Inside not so much. We have made the downstairs look sort of finished with a proper kitchen built especially for us, but not by us, which was a luxury. We are still using a ladder to get upstairs but with a shower and toilet downstairs, our guests need not be bothered by it. Finishing is going to be a very slow job indeed and we can't expect any more from the bank. They feel we have borrowed all we can against an unsellable asset.

Chapter 26: Baby Catching

"One of your patients has gone crazy and won't let the midwife into the room," the Delivery Suite Charge yells down the MHU hot phone. "You *have* to do something."

Firstly, all "our" patients are accounted for. I guess this is someone "known" to the MHU. If they are in the birthing unit then they are either in labour, or are a visitor and hampering someone who is.

Since I have the best qualifications – i.e., have given birth myself – I am voted to go. At least I'm not best dressed; birthing units can be messy places. The heavy MHU doors release me to the tranquillity of the corridor. I love hospital corridors; they serve as interludes between variants of pandemonia. Sometimes it isn't so much an escape, as dodgem, with meal trolleys, beds (with or without occupants), lost visitors, cleaners, and sundry emergencies, but when I exit the acute MHU today the wide, clean corridor feels like a sanctuary. Cool and silent.

If someone "known" to the inpatient unit is pregnant then we would not necessarily be privy to that information. Anyone who's been an inpatient on the MHU is perfectly entitled to break bones, have heart attacks, even get cancer without informing us. I am not sure staff on other units understand this. A large, angry Irish Charge Nurse greets me – she doesn't seem the sort to be messed with; she gives me the lady's name. Yes, I do know her, and I do know she is pregnant. I had no idea when she was due, but her sister lives in our village and she told me. At the time I had asked how she thought her sister would cope. She had suggested it could be the making of her; if not, then family would step in. So where is her support now?

Sandra is quite young; she must be about nineteen now. She came to the attention of the Mental Health Team as a fifteen-year-old, diagnosed with ambiguous disorders to fit the tick-box paperwork. It isn't uncommon; a significant number of teenage girls aren't right in the head, and no one wants to diagnose them with something that public perception believes is the end of the road. She has been given all manner of medication and in quite a combination. This is where I get angry. We have had forty years to do better. The pills that were supposed to fix everything can't replace skills and techniques to cope better with what life throws at you. But there aren't enough counsellors or psychologists. Pills are a band-aid for depressed and anxious teenagers, but Sandra's problems are at the scarier end of the spectrum, and without proper support her outlook isn't great.

The birthing unit is quite modern. It used to be part of the maternity ward but now they are split, and the birthing unit is painted grey and pink. It is supposed to be soothing, but it looks more like a gay battleship if you ask me.

There is a bunch of nurses and midwives huddled around a grey door – not a birthing room but an ordinary patient room. Sandra is screaming at them to stay out, but at the same time I can hear the screams of her labour. Not everyone screams. I poke my head around the door – she is standing, her legs apart. She instantly relaxes.

"Oh, it's you." She smiles. "Thank goodness you are here – I can feel the head between my legs. Can you catch?"

Oh shit, our schoolteacher always sent me as far out on the wing as you could get, and the team knew the ball should never come my way. I can sense some urgency though and I skid on my knees like a soccer player who's scored as the baby falls into my arms.

I've just delivered my first baby. It didn't even bounce! The audience breathes – clearly relieved. Now what the fuck do I do?

A young midwife sneaks through the door and slaps a clamp on the umbilical cord. I calm down a bit and Sandra lies on the bed. While the midwife does her thing, I distract Sandra by plonking the recently separated baby on her naked belly. She can work out the boy-girl dilemma; I would hate to get it wrong. I think this is enough for one day – but it seems my work is not yet done.

Sandra leaps up, dumping the baby on the bed. "I need a shower – NOW!"

She is off in a flash, with the cut and clamped umbilical cord hanging between her legs, the placenta retained. I follow her out of the room as the midwife scoops up the infant to check her over. Sandra runs to the shower, turns on the taps, and is straight in without checking the water temperature. The Charge assures me the placenta is safe enough for now, but just as she says it, Sandra removes the clamp.

The blood pumps from the cord with fair pressure behind it, and, in the confines of the shower it hits the wall and ricochets. Sandra has it in her hand, using it as some kind of terrifying hose, and it sprays everything in its path as it crosses the open door. Soaked in blood, I go to the kitchen and make a cup of tea.

"Bloody psych nurse – claret everywhere and she's making a cup of tea." I hear the Irish brogue.

She isn't wrong; I am taking a huge gamble, but I cannot risk fighting in a blood-soaked concrete shower cubicle. Walking past the bathroom with a tray of tea, I call out to Sandra, "Put the clamp back on – I have made us some tea. I'll take it to your room."

She replaces the clamp and follows like a lamb. We sit drinking tea and chatting about old times. She seems to have forgotten the baby, but in the back of my mind I know the placenta cannot stay where it is. I trust things are going on behind the scenes, and as we begin to run out of conversation a doctor arrives. He has exactly the reassuring presence needed for this situation. He explains what he is going to do. He doesn't give her alternatives, just a matter-of-fact description. "The placenta can't stay there. I am going to give you an injection. I will tug at it gently and it will come away."

She will be in theatre if it doesn't work, but we avoid any mention of that. His confidence makes her believe him and trust him. Everything works as he describes, and now she wants to sleep.

Apparently I'm a *bloody miracle worker*. You should never underestimate the power of a cup of tea. I escape while everything is quiet in case things kick off again.

I look like someone who narrowly escaped the Bates Motel. Better work stories, they said! The last couple of hours have been mental. This isn't going to be a good look back at the MHU, dripping with someone else's blood, but shopping in this state would have me arrested. I come up with a brilliant solution. The theatre is tucked away in the bowels of the hospital, and with endorphins kicking in after my first – and very likely only – delivery, I skip down two stairs at a time.

"Can I borrow some scrubs?"

They take one look at me, stuff me in a shower and throw my clothes in a washing machine.

I feel quite important in the green cotton scrubs, the closest I have ever come to wearing work clothes that are both practical and hospital funded. Of course, I know everyone in the MHU will take the piss out of me.

My next shift is the Friday night shift. I go in early to peek at "my baby". Things seem to be settling down, and as I wander through the silent corridors, I am hoping for a peaceful and blood-free shift.

I have done something astonishing for the girl of working-class parents, described by one teacher as a waste of oxygen. I am about to graduate with a Bachelor of Science, with a double major in biochemistry and molecular biology. It was on the bucket list. I don't come from an educated background; I have had to fight and squeeze it in bit by bit. So much of my study has been in the early hours of the morning when ordinary people are asleep. Yet since I finished the final exam at the end of last year – I have been restless. Now I have enrolled in a master's degree at The University of Auckland. Keep busy.

I manage to get extra tickets for the May graduation in Palmerston North, and my parents come to watch. It isn't the best time of year to holiday half-way around the world leaving one winter for another and we get snowed in at Ruapehu. I think they enjoy themselves and we squeeze in some tourist type things. We have managed to get the upstairs walls

226

covered in gib, not painted but they at least there is some privacy and Anthony sleeps on a linen shelf in Zach's room. He doesn't mind because it means his room is more finished than anyone's.

—◠◡◠—

The new unit is now being fully utilised so we have the locked ward back and now four night staff. The two units are symmetrical with a shared courtyard flanked on either side by bedroom wings. For some bizarre reason the end wall of the courtyard is a high concrete-faced wall. There is a glass slit at either end so you can see what a fabulous view you're missing out on. Each unit has a large lounge, dining room and kitchen, with a shared secure area. Each secure room has its own toilet and shower and a glass wall to an inaccessible garden. There's an office for each ward adjacent to the secure area with a short narrow corridor running between them, and the secure area can be accessed from either office or from either ward. The night staff are separated from one another by two doors. We generally prop them open; it seems mad not to be able to talk.

The decorating hasn't panned out the way we envisaged. Although we spent months agonising over colours and finishes, it hasn't got the colour, carpet nor lino we chose. Instead, it's been done on the cheap with something left over from elsewhere. A prison, I thought until the baby-catching incident; now I realise they must have had a job-lot of the grey from the birthing unit. It hasn't been lost on the patients – that wastage from elsewhere will do – for *those* people.

The apex of each lounge ceiling is easily six metres, and in my nightmares, I don't have time to do any masking or remove clocks or pictures – I simply speed-roll yellow paint, perhaps a relic from Stone House, around anything in my way so I can complete both lounges before I wake up.

—◠◡◠—

I have been called back in to do another transfer; it's a bit late in the day, but money for old rope. I know this guy; I don't consider him a threat at all. His is a sad story of someone who

227

never recovered from the death of a sibling. He is in A&E, having put his fist through a window with wired safety glass. Clearly not very safe because he has turned his fist into chips and done a huge amount of damage to ligaments, tendons and muscles, and it is wrapped up like a huge ball.

They did say he was sedated. He leaps off the trolley and runs out of the building. Heading downhill, I'm no shabby runner but he almost reaches the main road by the time I catch him; help isn't far behind. I do a flying leap tackle and feel something go in my wrist.

No time for fussing about; the ambulance is waiting, and we won't be back till the early hours as it is. They sedate him again and give me another injection to take with me in a brown paper bag. The accepting hospital is on the list of closing concerns, and run down, but my patient is happy there and the staff know him. It won't be a problem, but it is a long way, and it will take more than a shift.

Except it doesn't. We have lights and sirens, and at one point the back doors fly open, the paper bag flies out and we almost follow. This is because the door was not properly checked in the rush to leave, and the ambos are grumpy about stopping on the motorway to fix it.

Coming back isn't any better, and there was no need to rush in either direction. We make it there and back in six hours. This is the first time I have ever laid a complaint; the journey was unnecessarily terrifying. A&E tell me to come back in the morning if the wrist is still causing trouble. I smash through the gears in our van, trying to get home in the middle of the night with a scaphoid fracture in my left wrist.

—∿—

You never know what you're going to get with night shift. Sometimes it is absolute mayhem all night long. Other times you are bored senseless. I can't be doing with being bored so I always have something to do. I study – a lot, a bit like an expensive hobby. I still have the family newspapers to make. Occasionally I will read or knit but I can't watch TV or have a bit of a nod.

Sometimes I shoot the shit with my colleagues, and this night Mark and I are alone on the unit covering two wards while the others are at lunch. It is around 1:00 a.m., late enough to cast around for something to do to stay awake; the place has been silent all night.

Then Mark ripped a huge fart. He was rocking back on his chair, a big comfy thing he had dragged into the office from the lounge. You need to know something about Mark. He is around 6' 6". Slim, blond, good looking but he knows it. He turned up at a birthday party as a stripagram to the tune of "I'm Too Sexy". Still, he's a laugh.

Instinctively he reaches for his lighter to light the fart. The whoosh of flames takes both of us by surprise and he falls backwards. This is why your teacher tells you not to rock on your chair. The flames shoot along both his legs since they are now pointing skyward. I should somehow smother the flames, avoiding his crotch – he would dine out on that for ages. But then I see a pool of blood.

I am alone and responsible for the welfare of thirty-six mentally ill people, but my co-worker is unconscious, on fire and bleeding from a crack on the back of his head because he landed on one of the legs of the base of a wheelie office chair – his official chair. I'm not sure this situation was covered during my training. Midwifery, emergency triage and even firefighting were all sadly lacking. I throw the fire blanket over him. This is going to be a long shift – think of the paperwork alone!

Figure 7. Normal shoulder (not mine)

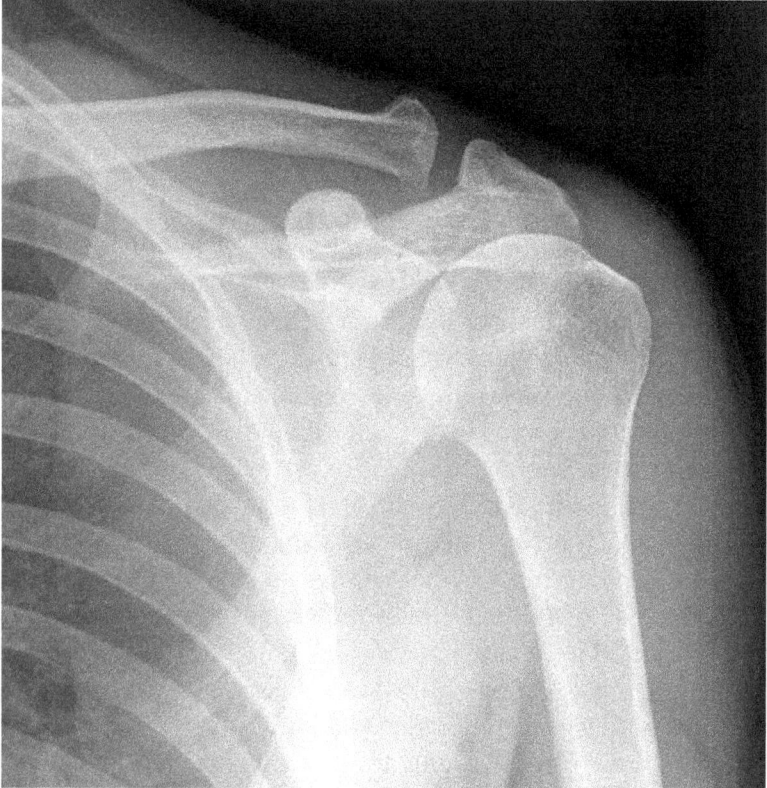

Credit: Gaillard F, 2025

Chapter 27: Terminal Times

A huge fight breaks out in the dining room. Nurses run from all around. Two of the clients have come to blows. They are called clients these days. It makes it sound as if they choose to avail themselves of our service. The young man who threw the first punch is detained under a court order.

Today's problem is that he believes the other lad has killed his parents, and he is determined to avenge their deaths. In a way it is touching to see the fire in his eyes demonstrating the love he feels for his adoptive parents. He is nineteen and muscular from years of farmwork since school proved unsuitable. The other lad is wiry but strong enough that some real damage is on the cards. It scares the willies out of everyone, and it takes six staff members to part the fighting pair. Someone calls the parents. No one is dead – they are on their way.

When there is an incident like this everyone is affected. The anxious are left in shock, the withdrawn retreat completely, and who knows what the confused and psychotic feel about it. The people who should organise a debrief are tied up with paperwork. Worse still for me – I am badly injured. It is collateral damage – I was caught between a body and a wall. Usually, I am the first person sent in to de-escalate a situation because I am the least threatening staff member. Some women will have a go at me; the lads take one look and realise their street credibility is down the drain if they lash out in my direction. Today, though, was beyond a few quiet words.

At last a sort of calm descends, and I slip out to X-ray – the paperwork can hunt me down.

X-ray is about as far away from the MHU as you can get, and to be honest I'm taking my time. My thoughts turn to the poor parents. Their lives revolve around their son; they have no choice. Some parents make a choice, and their offspring get what we call a geographic cure and end up here. It doesn't do much for the client – no friends, no family, and they don't even know where the local shops are (although this is much nicer place than some of the slowly emptying bins elsewhere). It suits the family though.

Last year a client died after jumping off a bridge. Earlier he'd been found dirty and dishevelled, living in the bush (though clearly lacking the skills and resources required for that kind of carry on). He had refused to give a name, though by the time he disappeared from our care we knew who he was. Nonetheless, he was identified by his fingerprints.

He had escaped through a broken bathroom window. I was not on duty, but in a mad way I feel responsible. The week before his escape a window in one of the doors to the courtyard had been broken during the night. I insisted someone come and board it up. I told the emergency maintenance man that otherwise I would have to call in a staff member on overtime to sit next to the broken window all night, which would be more costly than someone coming and nailing a bit of ply over it.

I was in so much trouble. But the thing is, I have to sleep at night (or day) and if someone had escaped or had used a shard of glass as a weapon, then it would have been down to me. It had to be fixed.

When the bathroom glass was broken the following week, the staff were understandably wary and left it. Our man took the opportunity to leg it and threw himself headfirst off an overpass.

All this thinking whilst strolling through the wide brightly lit corridors in actual agony is making me glum. To be fair, I don't think I'm firing on all cylinders.

My body is not broken, but it transpires I am fragile, with thin bones, narrow gaps and trapped nerves. My shoulder may need surgery. I should be happy because it could be worse, but I am in a world of pain. The advice is six weeks of light duties, and a drug called DF118 (dihydrocodeine).

My boss is wild, "I need people at the coal face with balls of steel, I don't need you prancing around on light duties."

I should be flattered... and not having balls, steel or otherwise, I feel valued.

He hasn't finished. "Who will they send? A couple of Siamese twins dressed in scrubs?"

This has happened already – a qualified Registered Mental Health Nurse was once replaced with two surgical nurses so terrified they couldn't be parted. The reality is I am unlikely to be replaced at all. As luck would have it there *is* a useful job I can do. The nurse in charge of preparing outpatients (they don't get called out-clients) that might be suitable for a new wonder drug for psychosis is in intensive care, having been run over by a truck or similar. So, for now I am to go home and take these painkillers, and next week I'll start my day job in the clinic. How hard can it be?

It turns out to be quite a cushy number. I make appointments for potential candidates for the drug. They must be physically and mentally assessed and have a sound understanding of the possible ill effects in order to provide informed consent. I organise a chest X-ray, do an EEG (electroencephalogram) – I had a cramming session with the instruction book since we didn't do this in my training! I sort paperwork, phone clients to see how they are, and organise the weekly blood tests and follow up appointments. Nothing stressful, nothing physical and all in daylight!

The drug in question is Clozapine (brand name Clozaril). To get on the trial a client needs to have treatment-resistant schizophrenia. That is, they have to have been trialled and failed on two or more traditional antipsychotics. This drug isn't even a new medication; it was shelved since the side effects were deemed to be serious and life threatening. Essentially it has been brought back by popular demand because it works.

It can cause a crash in the number of neutrophils (agranulocytosis). Neutrophils are a type of white blood cell that are especially important in fighting bacterial infections. That isn't the only problem; the drug can cause heart problems and constipation. Constipation might not sound like a big deal, but it kills more people on Clozapine than agranulocytosis.

The drug is not dispensed unless the client has an up-to-date white cell count.

I already know most of the clients since they have been on the unit at some stage. It is fabulous to see the total life change that occurs where the drug works well. These are people whose lives have been on hold and in some cases practically destroyed. They have been unable to hold onto jobs, relationships, even accommodation as their world crumbles away. Some are left vulnerable to unscrupulous people. Loved ones are left in despair.

—◢◣◢◣—

I have had three friends die in three days. Two from cancer, both far too young, and I lost a colleague and soul mate to suicide while I was on clinic duty. We both loved using odd words, I used to challenge him when I was away at university to use words like coprolalia in patients' notes.

I'm caught off guard by his death; I thought that if I had been on nightshift I would have known. There are plenty of male nurses in the mental health arena, but testosterone doesn't make them immune to those things that you wish you had never known. Sharing nightshift with someone, you get to know even their children's shoe size. There is more than a hundred years' experience amongst the six of us that make up the total contingent of the nightshift. Those lonely hours before dawn can make dark thoughts unbearable. But even with all that experience, no one foresaw the imminent suicide of one of our own. We were so wrapped up with everyday trauma, caring too much for too many.

On nightshift we would draw sofas on the evacuation chart to write the names of clients without a bed. Now in the hospital chapel I place a kiss on my colleague's forehead as he lies in his coffin; he succumbed to carbon monoxide in a hire car. He would have had the hire car in the hospital carpark all night.

—◢◣◢◣—

I could get used to light duties! Except the painkillers for my shoulder injury are messing with my head. I am not sleeping, and yet not really awake either. Sometimes I feel as if I am

234

watching myself from afar. I have the first-year exams for the MSc so on one hand it is helpful that I am not on shift work, but on the other I feel so far out of it.

"Like a tit in a trance," Stan says.

Then a blood test comes back from one of our success stories. A man in his mid-thirties, a cheerful and confident guy now living in a holiday park and getting his life back together, made possible by clozapine. I have a phone call of the worst kind to make. His neutrophil count is too low. He must stop taking the drug immediately. My fingers are shaking as I dial; this conversation must be intelligently handled.

I do my best, but the reaction is entirely as I expect. He is running through the traditional stages of grief.

"It's a mistake – you muddled up the blood tests." … "You bitch, how dare you do this to me." … "Let me redo the blood test. The next one will be good."

I try to negotiate my way through this but there is the sound of a car backfiring, so loud it must be right outside an open door. There is a long silence. The handset hasn't been hung back up on the receiver, but my client hasn't come back. I figure I can pop an appointment card in the post. This *is* important though; suppose he got an infection he couldn't fight while we're waiting for the post? The community team are less than twenty minutes from his address. I will see if someone is in the office – a friendly face at a time like this might help anyway. I can't recall if I phoned them or someone else did, it is blanked from my mind.

I am on leave from lunchtime. Tomorrow I will be in the wild with a heavy pack on my still sore shoulder, and in addition to the usual *everything but the kitchen sink* I will have a slab of cake and a bottle of wine. A friend of mine is running away from her own demons and enjoying an important birthday, tramping with me.

News filters back. He has blown off his head; it is smeared around the kitchen. I slide down the wall and sit on the corridor floor; the sound of the gunshot now ricochets around my brain.

For the last hour life has gone on as usual (not for him, obviously), and I had only been mildly anxious. There could be a hundred reasons for him leaving the conversation so abruptly. I am seemingly invisible on the corridor floor.

Today is the last day of the six-weeks' light duties following my shoulder injury. The painkillers have messed with my mind and to be honest the tramping holiday is my last hope. My deteriorating frame of mind from years of trauma and long hours has not been lifted by six weeks in a cushy number. In a recent and sudden abundance of caring by the senior management team, staff have access to the MHU psychologist. An anonymous survey reveals most of the team are clinically depressed; two should be compulsorily treated. I'm wondering why management think the unit psychologist is in any better shape than the rest of us. I know that trauma seeped into light duties long before my client blew his head off.

No one talks to me. There will be an enquiry, as if it will help with the here and now. No one has *ever* interviewed me as part of an enquiry.

I go home and stuff the wine and slab of birthday cake in my overladen pack. My friend turns forty by the time we near the end of the 46 km trek.

Everything is pinned on this adventure. Heavy pack, heavy heart and shoulder injury. I *have* been in this position before. When I was making up the missed time because of the car crash nothing had prepared me for the shock of giving a patient a routine injection and finding her dead not twenty minutes later. That day was the last day of my shift, and I faced days of not knowing. No cell phone in those days. The days were a blank.

Not much has changed, my phone doesn't ring.

Epilogue

New Year

My tramping holiday was supposed to fix everything. I was a fool for thinking it could. I lie in the hammock, the distant sound of fireworks welcoming in the new year. 1996 rolls over to 1997 to the sound of gunshot. It's seventeen years since my fateful decision to pay the bills by caring for others.

Consumer is the latest word of choice for a user of the mental health service. It sounds like someone is gorging on the system, I hate the word. Consumers have a voice, a choice in their care plan, and advance directives for future treatment. Psychiatry is no longer a dictatorship where your best interests are determined by someone else. Mostly this is a good thing but not if I think of Het (Henrietta) from my student days who had Huntington's chorea.

I think this is the worst way to die. Your mind and body cease to be under your control, you become paranoid and accuse others of malicious intent. It starts with your hands not doing as they are told. You can hide it at first, pretend you are sweeping back your hair as your hand randomly jumps at your face, but eventually you become unable to feed yourself as the spasms take over. That isn't the worst of it though. By the time you become aware of the symptoms, you already have children of your own and you have passed it on to half of them. Of course, you could have passed it along to all or none, such are the stats, a toss of a coin.

Het tried to refuse medication but she got it anyway – crushed up in her food so she never knew. As a result, her life or rather, her death, was a happier circumstance than that of a patient I nursed years later, George. No longer permitted to be duplicitous, we had to accept George did not want to take the medication we knew would ease his travails, and inevitably he suffered.

Darenth Park has closed, the Friern also; Mabledon closed, and the few remaining Poles have gone to Stone House.

237

Closure of Stone Hose has not been announced. It will close, of that I am certain, but thanks to the Grade II listing it won't be torn down – at least not all of it. Perhaps that's why it's still open: if it can't be removed then the land value is less. It will cost a fortune to bring it up to scratch, and for what purpose?

After six weeks of doing nothing I *must* go back to work; there are bills unpaid, some for a long time. I *was* adept at paying different people late each month so as not to piss the same person off all the time, but recently my head has been firmly in the sand. My sick pay is less than half my regular pay because although the Monday and Tuesday dayshifts were regular, they were never in my contract and therefore not in my sick leave. Penal rates for the early hours of Saturday went years ago in a pay *rise* that I never agreed to because for me it was a pay cut. We are scarcely managing; I'm not opening the bills.

I am drinking less tea – less anything – so I don't have to get up to pee. Stan is, of course, concerned. He has taken to coming home from work at lunchtime because he knows I won't have lunch unless he brings it to the hammock. He wishes I had a broken arm, something he can understand. He doesn't know why my heart can't feel any joy.

I used to love fireworks, immersed in the colour, the sound, the smell – especially the smell. It got lessened a little by learning that the colours are produced by electrons in the metal salts used in the manufacture of fireworks. The electrons get excited and jump to a higher energy level in a precisely known way. Then as they lose energy they fall back down, emitting a photon of light in a colour matching the lost energy.

It is the basis of spectroscopy. For instance, sodium streetlamps give off an orange light as their excited electrons fall back to ground state. Depending on the wavelength of the photon, we see a particular colour. I watch anyway, imagining the various metals in each firework – copper for green, strontium for red – but the similarity to the sound of gunshot is disturbing. And now everything is black and white, as if my mind has forgotten colour once existed.

The gunshot isn't the problem though – there is a petrol bill unpaid since May, before the suicide of my soulmate, before the suicide of my client. Patients have a voice, but nurses do not. Not one person has *ever* asked me what part I played in the demise or injury of a single soul. Wouldn't you want to know if you had done a wrong thing? If your practice could be improved?

During the last decades I have written a ton of incident reports. Does anyone read them? I am invisible and impotent. I no longer feel as though I can do anything. I have completed a double major in molecular biology and biochemistry in addition to my nursing qualification. Now I have started a master's degree. Yet I can't see how I can ever be of any use. The purpose of the master's degree is to validate my existence. I tell myself I am working towards my bucket list goals and in a way I am. I don't know why, but that list might be the only thing that will get me out of this hammock.

Having been thrown out of a good school at fifteen, a posh school by local standards, I have been playing catch-up. I wasn't the right student to make the most of the opportunity I had, and I prevented someone who deserved the place from having it. I wasn't mature enough to realise it. My parents made sacrifices to get me to the school I blew out of, and their disappointment weighs heavily.

Obviously, since then I have made study a priority in my life; no one goes from high-school drop-out to master's student without becoming a mega-nerd. The children have seen it. My study habits rub off on them, and they are all smart. I won't say they are all studious, but I am proud of them. I spent two entire semesters away from home. Without Stan to hold the fort none of it would have been possible.

Now my MSc is supposed to be preventing me from going barmy. And I need it before I can apply to become a doctoral student. I am in this for the long haul. I move from hammock to sofa in the evenings and eventually to bed but am back in the hammock by the early hours. Tonight is special. Since it is New Year, I might skip both sofa and bed.

New Year Celebrations

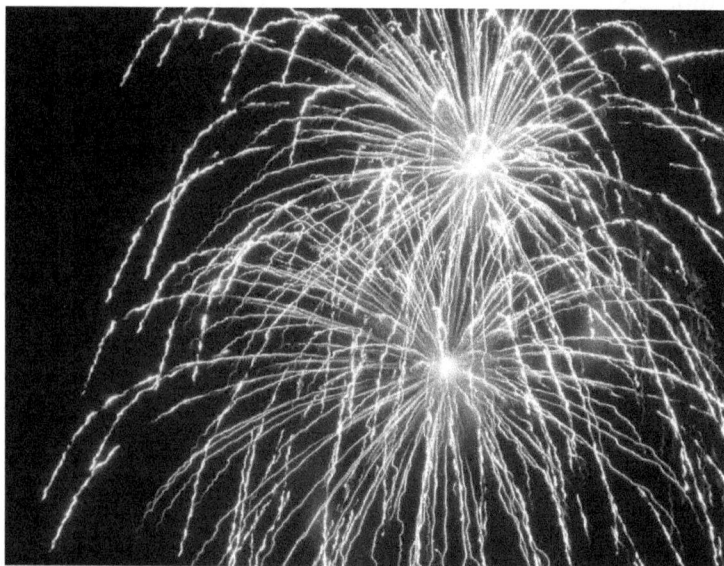

Personal photograph New Year Sydney 2013

Acknowledgements

The guy who pushed me out of the train should have stopped to see if I were OK. Around a hundred people died falling from those slam-door trains before they were withdrawn. I don't know who he was just as I don't know anything of the older woman who asked me how badly I wanted to study science. They were both pivotal to changes in my life. I think this counts as a butterfly effect. We don't know, how our actions will impinge on the future of someone else.

I had some fantastic Ward Sisters during my training, especially in Female admission at Stone House and the Mental Health Unit at Joyce Green. Without them I am sure I would have quit and I take my hat off to anyone who can do what they can. Now in New Zealand there are many talented and caring souls that made working in the MHU a happier time than it perhaps sounds, I thank you all.

My husband promised he would always prevent my ending up as a bag lady, and he has done so with diligence helped by my children who can mix it with anyone, their tolerance, patience, forgiveness and kindness to others and their encouragement of me is humbling.

I have had the support of NorthTec, as an employer, but also as a student of creative writing. I have tutors who always make me feel more talented than I have felt myself and over the years classmates have given support and critique in equal measure and made me a better writer.

My own students have also taught me many things. Most of them want to be nurses and I'm paid to help facilitate their dreams with a decent dose of chemistry and biochemistry. They don't always like it but we have fun and I try to give them an *out*. Nursing isn't for everyone. Mostly they ignore me but they will remember that I tried to caution their bright-eyed expectation with a dose of realism.

Mum has died and Dad has lost his marbles. I realise it is imperative that I write everything on what passes for paper or it will be lost.

Will the movies that play in my head cease when my marbles roll away? I hope so.

If you want to know what happened next, then *Bleak Expectations* will follow in 2026. If you are interested in my writing I have a blog https://lindykato.com/

References

Hole A, Terjesen T, Breivik H. (1980) *Epidural versus general anaesthesia for total hip arthroplasty in elderly patients.* Acta Anaesthesiol Scand. Aug;24(4):279-87. doi: 10.1111/j.1399-6576.1980.tb01549.x. PMID: 7468115.

Mental Deficiency Act 1913 - *Chapter 28* (The text of the Mental Deficiency Act 1913 was prepared by Derek Gillard November 2019) https://education-uk.org/documents/acts/1913-mental-deficiency-act.html

Figures

Figure 1. Watkins, J. (Illustrator) (1866). *The City Lunatic Asylum, near Dartford*. [Illustration]. The Illustrated London News. Held by the Wellcome Library London. File number L0004819. https://wellcomecollection.org/works/aq9wtcwb CC BY 4.0

Figure 2. *Unknown photographer from sales catalogue (circa 1965). Ectron series 3 electroshock therapy device.* [Photograph]. Agent Gallery https://agentgallery.com/objects/1960s-electroshock-therapy-unit

Figure 3. Jandhands (Photographer) (1988) *Darenth 6 "Not-forgotten Asylums in the UK"*. [Photograph]. https://www.flickr.com/photos/j_and_h/551923285/in/album-72157600364036452/

Figure 4. Powell, A. (Photographer) (1930). *Joyce Green Hospital, near Dartford*. [Photograph]. The metropolitan Asylums Board and its work, 1867-1930. Held by the Wellcome Library file number L0006810EB. https://wellcomecollection.org/works/pwf6hwsy CC BY 4.0

Figure 5. NIAID (2022) *Treponema pallidum Bacteria (Syphilis)*. [Electron micrograph]. https://www.niaid.nih.gov/news-events/niaid-syphilis-research CC BY 2.0.

Figure 6. Philafrenzy (Photographer) (2017). *The Friern Hospital*. [Photograph]. https://commons.wikimedia.org/wiki/File:Friern_Hospital_05.jpg CC BY-SA

Figure 7. Gaillard F, (2025) *Normal shoulder*. [Photograph]. Case study, Radiopaedia.org https://doi.org/10.53347/rID-7505 CC BY

www.ingramcontent.com/pod-product-compliance
Lightning Source LLC
LaVergne TN
LVHW041315080426
835513LV00008B/466